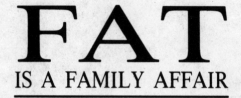

FAT
IS A FAMILY AFFAIR

FAT

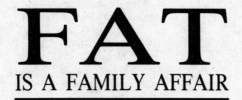

IS A FAMILY AFFAIR

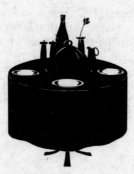

JUDI HOLLIS, Ph.D.

A Hazelden Book
HarperCollins*Publishers*

ISBN: 0-06-255434-4

Printed in the United States

92 93 94 FAIR 16 15 14 13 12

Editor's Note:

Hazelden Educational Materials offers a variety of information on chemical dependency and related areas. Our publications do not necessarily represent Hazelden or its programs, nor do they officially speak for any Twelve Step organization.

TO HOPE

"Beyond a wholesome discipline,
be gentle with yourself. . . ."

Desiderata

Acknowledgments

Yves Luc Bolomet is my editor, companion, best friend and seer, but most of all, he's the "Prince Charming" I was not ready for until I grew up. He's taught me equality, respect, and how to love. As professional mentors, William Ofman, Ph.D. taught me the "good faith" of honest relating, while Walter Kemplar, M.D. showed me how to move whole families along the journey to intimacy, and Bill Rader, M.D., throughout our long and varied association, encouraged the wisdom of "trusting your instincts."

My deepest appreciation and joy go to the thousands of patients and counselors who have shared the hope of their recoveries. It is a humbling privilege that they allow me into their lives. Thanks to my dad, Gilbert Stockman, who expected me to be a full person, and my mother, Rebecca Stockman, who showed me the strength I'd need. Special thanks go to Elaine Goodrich who listened to my inner voice until I could hear it myself. Thank God for the Twelve Steps.

Contents

Introduction

"We're as fat as we are dishonest"

Fat is a family affair, because we've all been living with a dishonest person who sought to survive by living a lie. To win love and admiration, we acquired an "as if" personality, becoming what others needed and losing a sense of inner self. When that true person cried out to be heard, we drowned it out with food. Recovery from an eating disorder requires a precious journey to find the real self. Most of us are unable to find the way on our own because we wear blinders when forks loom up in the path. It is easier to trudge the well-beaten, painful path than to risk the unknown.

Loved ones have helped us live the lie as they live out their own. As long as we keep eating, we can ignore internal messages that say, "Something is wrong with my life." I was a very successful therapist at 222 pounds, and had no idea that anything about my lifestyle was at all related to the poundage I'd amassed. I actually thought I was a nearly perfect human being—my only minor flaw was the fat. If I'd lose weight, I'd be perfect and so would my life. I'd lost thousands of pounds before, as a college freshman on pills, then each of the nine times at Weight Watchers, as well as countless other failed attempts. Each time, despite a gorgeous body, nothing had changed in my personality. I still felt inadequate despite a false bravado, and I still never felt deserving of the good life, and couldn't endure the stress of success. Slowly the weight crept back.

This time has been different. I've not only kept the weight off for over nine years, but I lost my childish demands to be rescued and found the very wise, sensitive, and real adult I'd been drowning. I had to be reborn and become a baby first. Then I could grow up without food. As a result, I had to renegotiate every relationship in my life and establish a new identity for success.

To recover from an eating disorder we have to give birth to the true self, find a way for it to be heard, then carry it with us into a new life. The most healing and long-lasting method for gaining such a recovery is taught at meetings of Overeaters Anonymous. Through that program and suggestions in this book, you can find a new way to RELATE TO RECOVER.

The body doesn't lie. The head may talk us into things or convince us to accept the unacceptable, but our body's deformity graphically shows how much we are out of kilter with our true selves. Our culture teaches us to respect or reject the self using false standards. How can anyone feel okay wearing size twelve when Madison Avenue says to wear size five? We usually settle for size 24 and give up the struggle. Eating is a substitute for true intimacy and risk. If we want to change our bodies, we have to change our relationships. Whether bingeing, vomiting, or starving, an eating disorder is a symbol or symptom of how we relate in the world. Overeaters, anorexics, and vomiters all have this in common. Whether 50 pounds underweight, 300 pounds overweight, or struggling with the same fifteen pounds daily for years on end, each sufferer must examine the same issues of control and vulnerability.

We have tried to get nurturance without being vulnerable. The only way to do that is with food. Food is that single, solitary, lonely substance that is ever ready and never fails. Food never expects anything of us. We don't have to entertain it with small talk and we don't even have to take a shower for it to love us. People aren't quite that predictable or dependable. People sometimes expect too much. Refusing to risk the pain of separateness from others, we choose the controlled security of food. Eventually the food itself becomes uncontrollable. Then we must give up food and return to others. This affects everyone in our lives. This book is for you and all of them.

Renegotiating relationships is much harder than fasting or gulping down water coolers. You might be turned off to this approach as too hard. You already know the other "quickie" books don't work. They're tossed in your bedroom corner with the Snickers wrappers. For you the question must be, "Do I want to have another quickie just this once, or do I really want to get on with it, once and for all, whatever it takes?" It's a clear and personal choice. You don't even have to take care of it in *this* lifetime. Whatever growth you are avoiding will still be waiting for you the next time around.

Denying your true self left you irresponsible. You avoided responsibility for yourself and others. A fat buffoon threatens no one, and if you keep failing, no one will expect too much. Neither will you. This book is about taking yourself seriously and gaining respect from yourself and others. Your life is at stake. You have nothing to lose but your fat.

As I sent this book proposal to a number of publishers, I was overwhelmingly rejected with, "The approach is too serious." Here is some of what I was told:

"A very thorough proposal and an excellent book idea. The trouble is, I think, that most people want a quick, new diet program that works for them. So while a book for behavior modification for the whole family and or friends makes some sense, I don't think it can compete with those other books."

"My experience with books having to do with eating disorders is that the more serious they are the less well they sell and that books that don't provide diets don't sell at all."

"Unfortunately, as we all know, the diet books that work are the 'magic' books, and while they may not be healthy, they offer people what they want."

"*Fat is a Family Affair* is not only *not* a diet book, but one which requires a great deal of time and effort on the part of the person who suffers from the problem, and from the family members as well. In other words, I think it's just too much work."

"*Fat is a Family Affair* could be the hottest diet book since sliced pineapple and papaya and still I'd think it was chopped liver!"

I take pride and compliment in the words of my detractors. If those are the reasons for rejecting this manuscript, I offer them to you, the reader, as a tribute to your dedication to finally take on the difficult task. As we joked in high school when asked to try something new, "May as well, can't dance. . . ."

Judi Hollis, Ph.D.

THE WEIGH IN

Chapter One

Relate to Recover

I was never truly thin until I grew up and became an adult. I had lost weight before, but I'd never grown up before. I had been married and divorced and was still looking for a "big daddy" out there to "fix" me. That was years after I had lost and gained thousands of pounds, but, emotionally, I did not know how to be independent and responsible to myself. I had mistaken senses of responsibility; I tried to prove my worth by helping others, but I didn't know how to heal me. I ate! I was a living dress rehearsal. That is, in part, why I became a therapist. I hoped that by delving into why I ate, I would one day be able to stop eating compulsively. Life would begin when I got thin. I also hoped that helping others would heal me by osmosis. Regrettably, these plans did not work. I found that helping others drained me, and intense therapy only left me lonely and depressed. So I did what any compulsive overeater would do—I ate. It was a roller coaster: gaining, losing, bingeing, abstaining, examining, ignoring, and, ultimately, eating.

Even though eating became a larger and larger part of my life, I did manage to develop a career. Professional success helped hide my bingeing. I was certain hiding it would make it vanish. However, I became fatter and fatter and my "secret" became more and more obvious.

I was a gifted teacher and trainer in the addiction counseling field. I lectured internationally about the problems of addiction for heroin abusers and alcoholics. Just before stepping on stage, I would agonize about my posture and appearance. I contorted like a twisted pretzel to keep the bulges from showing. Sometimes I would actually binge before a lecture to gain enough security to speak. At one international congress, I even burped at the end of my speech, punctuating the buffet of an hour before.

My bulges weren't the only thing to hide. While I was lecturing, I also kept secret the fact I was married to a practicing alcoholic. Despite all my best efforts, I could not fix him either. I had helped so many other families, but my own life was in shambles. The stronger the facade I projected, the more I kept falling apart. One thing kept me strong enough to keep up the front—food.

It was very easy to counsel and help alcoholic families, but impossible to see myself in the same fix. Colleagues marvelled at how well I worked with the addictive personality. They felt I had a natural gift for understanding alcoholic patients. Not one of them ever made the connection that I was just as sick and pained as the people I helped. I know now that my true illness was the denial of my own neediness masked by the service of helping others. We all denied the severity of my illness. After all, although alcoholism certainly seemed severe and deadly, we all assumed my problem was merely a struggle of willpower, and as soon as I mustered enough of old Will's power, I would pull myself up and do something. I always assumed that I would do it on a Monday. (We always binge on the weekends.) I showed a strong facade as a therapist, while I denied my own painful obesity. "Knowing it all" for my clients certainly didn't help me.

One September afternoon I walked past a store window and saw a horribly fat reflection in the glass. She wore a dress exactly like mine. It stopped me cold—the wind was knocked out of me. I stared fixedly into the glass and, somewhere deep within, a small voice whispered, "That lady in the window is *you.*" I could not speak or move! I was transfixed as I realized that my self-destructive journey was every bit as deadly and uncontrollable as any alcoholic's I'd ever treated. With all my best efforts, I weighed 222 pounds! I had *dieted* myself up to that weight. I had not done it by willy nilly eating. My life consisted of brief periods of controlled eating followed by excessive well-deserved bingeing. Dieting always began with firm resolve, clenched teeth, and white knuckle abstinence. When the pain of living without food became unbearable, I was soon back with my tried and true comforter.

I saw alcoholics who kept alcohol at bay by finding nurturance among people. I had been counseling them and their families into A.A. and Al-Anon for years. It suddenly seemed axiomatic that the cure for compulsive eating must follow a similar course. It might even be harder for overeaters; they had to control their substance daily. However, the fact that it was difficult didn't make it impossible.

That "impossible" feat, abstaining from compulsive eating, has been accomplished by myself and thousands of others with the plans described in this book. I have developed hospital treatment programs over the past decade helping overeaters, undereaters, and their families. The hardest part is acknowledging how hard it is and accepting help. If we could have done it on our own, we would have.

To recover from an eating disorder involves turning away from the self-administered comfort of food and turning instead to nurturance from people. Although my experience has been primarily with people seeking help in hospital treatment programs or private therapy, these are not the only avenues open. The crucial issue is admitting your own personal vulnerability. Once you can allow yourself to ask for help, you are well on the road to recovery. I have found that Overeaters Anonymous works best for the greatest number of people. This book will show you how to accept help and make Overeaters Anonymous work for you. You will see that as your personality changes, other people in your life will be adjusting to the changes and they will need help as well. Family members will learn how to get help from others and remove from themselves the burdens and expectations for a cure.

You may say, "But this will take too long! I might be forty before I'm thin." Well, you're going to be forty *anyway!* And you may stay thin for more than half an hour. These results will be longer lasting and you won't want to return to compulsive eating. You'll feel better with abstinence than you ever felt bingeing. There's nothing so bad that a binge won't make it worse.

We're going to mess up your food. You won't be able to eat in the same old way anymore. You will be too conscious of what you are doing. That very issue is the focal point of this recovery program. Your dishonest relationships with loved ones helped you deny and kept you fat. You were able to isolate from others as long as your friend, food, filled your needs. When you give up the food (and by this I mean your old attitudes and behaviors toward it), you will give up defiance, and you will need to get nurturance from others. When you learn how to get needs met from other people, the craving for food diminishes. In other words, you won't work on the food, but on the relationships. Your new neediness will affect every person you know, and this is what makes fat a family affair.

In recovery, eating disorder sufferers (E-Ds) and their codependents will change their relationships. In this book you will see who is an E-D and who is a codependent, and their interdependent relationships. E-Ds can be fat or thin; it is the obsession with food and control which predominates. Codependents can be near relatives or distant friends; the need to be helpful is controlling their lives. For each, new ways of relating will lead to recovery.

FOOD AS LOVE

Loving food is safer than loving people. This certainly sounds like a crazy idea! "What does one thing have to do with the other?" you wonder. They have everything to do with each other. Food and people are most intimate forms of caring. Actually, *eating is the most intimate experience any of us knows*. Think about it. When you take food into your body, you are bringing a foreign substance across your own personal boundaries and incorporating it into your very being. When you eat, the "outside" enters your own personal temple, juices from your own body mix with it and use it to make new cells! The food changes form and becomes new parts of you! Not even sexual intercourse involves such an intimate merging. This is total union. Seeking that total union and intimacy, we turn to food because people don't work as well.

BABY WANTS A BOTTLE

While still in the womb, you felt secure. You couldn't really separate where you began and mommy ended. It was safe, and life required very little effort. You never had to ask for a thing. The world anticipated your needs before you even knew what they were. You were full and safe without even knowing the possibility of feeling differently.

When the nurturing, effortless environment was disturbed by birth, you had to get out there and LIVE! Suddenly, you became an infant. As an infant, you experienced the differentness between you and the world. Much of your early development involved reaching for your own toes. You learned the difference between touching *your* toes and touching someone else's wooden crib. There *was* a difference. You also learned that sometimes *you* felt different inside. Sometimes you felt full inside and sometimes you felt empty. When you felt the emptiness, you didn't like it, so you cried and someone else fixed it. It may have taken a few minutes, but sooner or later Mom came, bottle poised, ready to fill your needs. "What took you so long," you wondered, "between the time when *I* knew I needed something and you fixed it? Why did I even have to cry? Why didn't *you* know what I needed? Isn't the rest of the world inside my skin? I don't like these delays! I definitely don't like the EFFORT it takes to live out here; it's a hell of a lot of work. . . ."

"THANKS A LOT, I'D RATHER DO IT MYSELF"

Since you learned early that it would require effort and might even sometimes be difficult, you decided to find another way to get your needs met. Other people are usually disappointing. Consider this a minute. Other people can't help being "wrong" for you. They are going to be having their own bad days. They have their own needs they're trying to meet. And, most important, they are not inside your skin; they can't anticipate your needs and save you from the effort of speaking.

Your decision to develop an eating disorder actually had some wisdom. It saved you from the painful realizations and disappointments that accompany the difference between you and other people—the reality that *they* may not be there for you. Since you felt you could not weather those disappointments, you decided to nurture yourself without *them*. That's what bingeing does. You are totally secure and safe while bingeing. Your need for nurturance is being met at a steady pace and you are totally in control of food. You buy it, prepare it, and devour it. That makes you totally self-sufficient. You don't need anyone else. In fact, when you are alone with food, you don't think of anything else, you feel at one with the universe. The separation is gone. There is a continuous motion between your elbow's bend and your jaw's chewing, and the precision of the act is perfection. The world is yours.

The anorexic, while refusing to binge, carries the self-nurturance even further. With anorexia, you are saying, "Not only don't I need YOU, I don't even need FOOD. I am so self-sufficient, invincible, invulnerable, and self-contained I can live on air. I have overcome any 'human' (said with a sneer) neediness and am completely in charge of my life. I'm *not needy!*"

Each is a way to feel in control and protected from the need for love. To avoid disappointment, you transfer all your neediness to an unnatural love affair with food. There's really nothing inherently destructive or problematic about this decision until carried to extremes. Although your case may not be extreme, it is your unnatural relationship with food and the use of it to avoid human nurturance that makes you an E-D. You are using food to avoid the risk of life. In this book you will learn how to risk life to give up food.

You will learn ways to risk showing the world exactly who you are and of turning to other people to help you. You will learn how to express your needs and feel grounded. Too often you ate to amass body size so you could feel solid. When you discover independence, you won't need all that flesh to prove you exist. The only freedom from the obsession with food is a new, healthier dependency on other people instead. People with broken legs use crutches, and people with eating disorders can turn to other people instead of food.

GIVING UP MEANS GROWING UP

Whether you are anorexic or obese, your decision to deny your own neediness and seek solace in food is a way to stay in control, albeit suffering. Staying focused on the food has been a way to avoid growing up and accepting the reality that *they* can't fix it. Maybe they should, but they can't. They can aid, but they can't fix! As a demanding, disappointed child you have proclaimed, *they* should be different. *They* should be there for me. *They* are trying to hurt me. Since *they,* (Mommy, Daddy, spouse, friend, employer) failed, you turn to a substance to keep filled and safe with the fantasy that instant gratification and a fix will always be there. Rather than face the disappointment that you might not be cared for well enough, you decided to do it yourself.

This is a survival mechanism. Perhaps your childhood was spent being your own parent, or parent to your parent. This is often true if born to an addicted family. Your addicted parent certainly could not be there for you, so you learned to do it yourself. Whatever the causes, you came by the decision to binge quite honestly. If your decision is to starve, you still have the same motivation. Usually, if anorexic, you started out with a weight problem (food to excess) and now seek to control the problem. The obsession with food once worked, but now it's turned on you. In any event, the way out is to face the disappointment. First, food has failed you, you can't control it. Second, people have failed you, they don't anticipate or meet your needs fast enough. Facing such disappointments is a way to grow up. So, they do fail you, now what? How can you still turn to others knowing they might sometimes fail you? You will have to learn to shop around. You will have to learn or eat. It's that simple. In recovery you will grow up with enough strength to know that others can care, but can't fix.

Families and friends need more help with this than the eating disorder sufferer. You will learn what a "codependent" over/under-eater is, and how much you want to rescue those you love from the painful reality of growing up and facing disappointment. In zealously rescuing them from disappointment, you have contributed to their problem and certainly not helped yourself. The best way to help them will be to start helping yourself. Living and facing life honestly is the road to recovery. Sometimes you are honestly fed up with rescuing. It's time to say that, and then stop doing it.

A crucial struggle is for parents and children to separate with love. The relationship of parent and child has to be severed and then slowly soothed and healed into something new. As long as parents feel overly responsible for their child, the child will not grow up and face life on its own. This separation is not just a matter of age or geographics. It is a deep emotional commitment and tie which must be broken for survival to occur. Sometimes the dependence is carried to a mate. You marry into a situation where you still believe someone else will fix you. As long as you both believe and perpetuate the myth, obsession with food will continue.

In order to grow up, you will have to change that very important relationship with food. As your most significant love object, food serves as both nurturer and punisher. It works when all else fails. It helps mask all your neediness and helps you avoid your own life. Most importantly, it helps you weather the stress of change.

It plants you firmly in concrete so you won't ebb and flow with the tide of life. Without the binding security of food, you will acquire the flexibility to flow with changes in your life.

FOOD AS AVOIDANCE

You have used food to avoid. With food you avoid

- the risk of knowing how much you need other people.
- the possibility that you won't have the world as you'd like it.
- taking responsibility for your own life.
- the probability that if you really wanted to, you could be ecstatically happy most of the time.
- the reality that even if life is great, there will also be bad days.
- the reality that *they* are not in your skin.

You must learn to change an unnatural relationship with food into a new relationship with others. Food will become cardboard. It is only a substance to stoke your engine for a 24-hour period. It is not love, sex, God, or rock and roll—it is just food.

And you are just you. You may not be all the things you or others planned you'd be, but you certainly are someone to yourself. This is your life, and your responsibility is to live it. Food keeps you away from the fullness of your life. You may be drowning in esoteric discussions of self-worth and personal image. What does it all have to do with anything? What is self-worth? Does a chair have worth? A table? It's only worth is in how you use it. Do you have use for a table? Do you have use for your life? It's here for you to enjoy. With the food obsession out of the picture, you'll be able to see what you've got.

FOOD AS PUNISHMENT

Maybe you can't enjoy life because you think you should be punished. You may be confused about nurturance and punishment. Mothers, in addition to being our chief nurturer early in life, are also our chief socializers. Mom teaches us how to adapt to our culture and fit in with the environment. Noted psychiatrist, R. D. Laing has quipped that "the Stone Age baby is born to the twentieth-century mother and that's where the process of violation begins." At birth you possess the same genetic programming and the same potentials bred into the savage Stone Age baby. However, you were born into a society where Stone Age behavior is not appropriate. Your mother's job was to teach you to survive in this culture. Some of your savage behavior had to be corrected and modified. You were told no, and you felt deprived; there was conflict between your wants and society's dictates. You received punishment and nurturance from the same source, so you are confused about what is nurturance and what is punishment. Food became your punisher as well as your solace. By the time you have picked up this book, it is difficult to sort out what is what. You may think you eat to get soothed, whereas you actually binge to punish yourself.

WE ARE *HOW* WE EAT

Food has been the major tool you've used in coping with life. To know who you are, just watch how you eat. Do you see yourself as a lady or gentleman sitting down to a genteel leisurely meal in a serene state of mind with classical music and place mats? Instead, are you in a garbage-strewn car with straws and wrappers and crumbs stuck in the cushions?

Eating with a driven frenzy, whether it is the pizza you obsessed about all day or the spontaneous decision to guzzle at the kitchen sink, is compulsive eating. Eating compulsively is a measure of your anxiety and inability to weather the frustration and stress of the life you are living. Food takes the shaking away. It seems to relieve the stress and helps you cope. Some may balk at this idea and fancy themselves as secure, independent, extremely competent individuals. They reject the idea that eating frenzies have anything to do with stress. They might even deny they have lives totally fashioned around showing how well they can manage and handle things.

That was certainly true in my case. At my top weight I was helpful to and needed by a lot of people. How could I believe that I was also needy? The food kept me from having to admit that fact. The only way you will find out how truly needy you are is when you stop eating compulsively. Until you stop the behavior, all your ideas about why you eat will be philosophical conjecture with no basis in life experience. I surely thought seeking the *why* of my behavior would be the way out. I studied and became a therapist in order to figure out why I ate. I found many reasons. Some were quite depressing, and *I ate over them*. What else could I do? The only way to see reasons for your behavior is to stop it first. Then you will be able to observe what develops. If you want to find out why you eat compulsively, don't eat compulsively. With little effort on your part, when the eating stops, your life will emerge. In other words, without the excessive feeding and the obsessional frenzies around food, whatever you have been submerging about yourself and your life will automatically bubble up.

In my case, I found I was scared to death to appear on the TV shows I had binged my way through. As I continued to curtail my eating behavior, I had to give up some of my consulting work. I was a workaholic and food helped me succeed and achieve. However, the price became too great. The more I made abstinence the number one priority in my life, the more clearly I saw that my life had to change. This had gradual but dramatic effects on the total personality I was to become without food as the base. I stopped punishing and learned how to savor the good life.

Whoever you think you are is who you have become *with food*. You really don't have any idea yet who you might be without food. That new person will gradually emerge as you give up the food. You'll see. So will your family and friends.

EAT TO LIVE OR LIVE TO EAT

If you eat only when hungry you certainly don't have any need to examine your life as a way to change your relationship with food. You are obviously only using food to stoke your engine for a 24-hour period. You are not obsessing about food or overindulging to relieve stress. This is true for my little dog, Samson. He lays around most of the day. He feels secure about his life. He has very few performance expectations for himself or from others. He's content. He can leave a bowl of food sit all day if his body doesn't call for it. He often leaves half his bowl and returns later to finish. I've even known humans like this. I might invite them to eat, and they'll refuse seconds saying something like, "No thanks, I'm full."

I always wonder, "What does hunger have to do with it? Don't they see what good stuff is here? Why do they push away a half-eaten plate?" They eat like my dog. Their eating is a natural life function, like breathing. Their attitude toward food is, "I'll take it when I have to, but I really don't care much about it either way." Can you imagine? They don't need this book. They eat to live.

And then there are those of us who live to eat. If you fall into this category, you spend a large part of your time thinking about and taking in food. You have adapted your life so that feedings fit casually into your schedule. Usually, you don't even know when you are eating. Filling yourself and feeling sedated has become an integral part of your life. It helps you handle feelings and needs that you might have judged as too excessive. Let's look at some of those needs, as recovery will involve finding a way to get those needs met without food.

Appreciation.　Rodney Dangerfield laments, "I don't get no respect." He's also fat. What about Jackie Gleason as Ralph Kramden who struggled to make Alice listen to him? Also fat. Often the fat person has colluded with those who don't respect him by making a joke of himself before anyone else can. Even so, eating is a way to assuage the disappointment at not being appreciated. Many women start to gain weight soon after marriage. After the romance and excitement of the wedding settle down, the bride stops getting all those pats on the back and appreciative best wishes. Hubby doesn't profess his love and devotion as often as he used to. If home is her only life and she isn't getting some of her strokes from the job, marriage can quickly lead to the comfort of food. Similarly, if the strokes from work aren't forthcoming, both men and women sometimes handle the disappointment by turning to food.

The excessive weight gains after childbirth have been explained as metabolic. They also have a lot to do with lack of appreciation. Unrealistic expectations of what the birth of the baby would do for your life result in disappointment and even depression after the delivery. One closely guarded secret is a mother's disappointment after the birth of a child. It is hardest for these young mothers to admit to themselves, that maybe it's not the big deal it was cracked up to be. It is difficult to speak openly about this. All the relatives and friends are fluttering around oohing and aahing. How could you possibly complain when everyone is telling you how happy you are? All kinds of presents and well wishes come from near and far for the new infant. Who sends presents to the mother? She's supposed to get enough joy and enough of a present just by holding the new baby. Where is there a place for her to say, "Oh my God! What have I done to my next twenty years? Where do I get mine?" The easiest solution is, "on the plate."

When the mother does accept the birth of the child with joy, she then dedicates herself to raising it well. After twenty-odd years, if she's done a good job, the infant leaves the nest. Again, "Where's mine?" With much discussion of the empty nest syndrome and women's needs for fulfillment, little specific attention has been paid to the mother's need for appreciation. In treating menopause, hormones are prescribed when a few pats on the back might do wonders. It is no accident that most of the women alcoholics who enter treatment do so in their 40s. Many women who don't cover up their needs in a bottle do it by overeating.

In recovery you will learn how to identify your need for appreciation and turn to people who can congratulate and applaud you as needed. By the time your covering up with food has progressed to its excessive stages, you may need appreciative pats on the back, not just from one or two people, but from crowds of people, a whole group. You need to be cautioned not to "take your bucket to empty wells." You may tend to insist and demand that you get those appreciation strokes from the very person who can't give them. This is very self-defeating. For example, the mother whose nest is being abandoned may demand that the adult daughter who is struggling to break away be the one to show her appreciation. This is a no-win situation. In order to make the break, the daughter may have to rebel and reject before she can later be ready to appreciate. The mother may instead need to turn to other mothers to help her be appreciated. Similarly, the daughter can't get support from the mother she is leaving. She will need to turn to other daughters for appreciation of her struggle.

I experienced this struggle for appreciation in my professional work. I worked with a famous psychiatrist who served as my mentor and a very strong influence on my life. I wanted appreciation and respect from him at the same time I needed to grow up professionally and move out from under his protective wing. He also needed appreciation for all he had taught me. We were both needy as well as strong. Unable to receive from one another, we each had to turn to others for support in weathering the separation. In my case, I had to seek out other appreciative supporters or return to the comfort of the plate.

Approaching the New. Newness and change can be terrifying. Instead of acknowledging and weathering the discomfort of new situations, many simply assume false bravado and plunge in with both hands and a knife and fork. Without food, you may have to feel the threat and challenge of new situations. At a party, you may have to feel the awkward shyness you have on first meetings instead of staking your ground at the buffet table and cracking a thousand jokes. On the job, you may have to sit back and learn more before showing off your brilliance and then running to the cafeteria. In other words, slow down and wait. You are right to be cautious and a little apprehensive in new situations. Let yourself feel the fear of change. Let the threat of the new come to the surface and then it can pass. Denying the threat of the new will keep you in the old. This is especially true if the change is for something better and more positive than you knew before. It will be harder to weather changes for the better.

Relaxation. Much eating is a way to relax and settle the tensions of life. At most jobs, a coffee break is acceptable and allowed, whereas twenty minutes of quiet meditation seems self-indulgent. Instead, you binge at your desk. Eating, anxiety, and work are tied together. You may often judge your needs to be alone and quiet as too withdrawn, isolating, when, in fact, you need the separation in order to regroup and listen to your own inner voice. When that voice isn't heard, it wants to eat.

Habit. Some eating is simply habitual as a tried and true response to various life situations. You expect to eat when the clock strikes noon whether you are hungry or not. Certain events evoke nostalgic feelings about certain foods. Rarely do you give yourself a chance to decide whether you really wanted to eat turkey on Thanksgiving or not. What about eggs for breakfast? Is that really what you wanted to eat, or do you eat eggs out of habit? Sometimes certain friends awaken cravings for certain foods. My friend Jennifer and I used to call each other up and say, "Wanna go 'porkin'?" This meant we would hit both Baskin-Robbins and See's candy and ride around in the car until we were nauseous. For many years in recovery, it was difficult for us to get together without craving a return to our habitual relationship. We had to learn new activities or else give up the friendship.

Sexuality. Have you ever described a hot fudge sundae as orgasmic? Much sexual energy is sublimated into licking ice cream cones and slurping puddings. With recent changes in women's roles, larger groups of women complain that they feel much more sexual and horny than their macho male partners. This is threatening in a culture previously based on male dominance and women's coy submissiveness. Guilty over such sexual feelings, many women have decided to become fat rather than sexually demanding. Their fat is then used by the man as the reason for his lack of interest. During the woman's recovery, these men feel threatened when the weight comes off and the excuse is removed. The relationship has to be renegotiated. When the option to eat the sundae is removed, you may experience tremendous sexual urges. Try not to be afraid of these, but accept them as what you have been pushing down with the food.

Competition. Much angry energy is put into achieving and pushing ahead. For many, your potential was almost fatal. Trying to accomplish and achieve much more than humanly possible, you often let yourself relax and calm down with a Snickers bar or a bag of Fritos. These munchy, crunchy foods are a way to express the rage. You give your mouth a chance to gnaw on your perfectionistic standards for yourself and others. In recovery, you find other ways to express your anger that are not so self-defeating.

Coping. Your major coping mechanism has been on your plate. You have not learned the other tools necessary for survival. Yours have been inadequate responses to life situations as a way to fill your need to please and manipulate others as well as a way to cover up your feelings of inadequacy and low self-worth. In recovery you will find a form of self-acceptance where you will feel whatever you can accomplish will have to be enough. Do the best you can and aim for progress, not perfection. You will be able to live with others' expectations as well as your own.

USING FOOD TO COPE IS DISORDERED EATING

If you cope with life through food you are probably suffering what has recently been labeled an eating disorder. In this book we will refer to you as an E-D. In the next chapter you will learn more specifically about medical diagnosis of your condition, but for now, please answer the following questions to determine the actual level of food abuse in your life.

Let's see if you are an E-D. An E-D is someone who is obsessed with food and dieting. You may be fat or emaciated. Food has assumed unnatural importance in your life and has come to dominate you, both psychologically and physically.

E-D QUESTIONNAIRE

	YES	NO
Do you feel guilty about eating?	___	___
Are you prone to consume large quantities of junk food?	___	___
Do you hide food or hide from others while eating?	___	___
Do you eat to the point of nausea and vomiting?	___	___
Are you sometimes repulsed by food?	___	___
Do you relish preparing foods even if you don't eat?	___	___
Have you forced vomiting?	___	___
Do you take many laxatives to control weight?	___	___
Do you weigh in on a scale more than once a week?	___	___
Have you found yourself unable to stop eating?	___	___
Have you taken on fasting to control weight?	___	___
Do you know your eating pattern is abnormal and embarrassing?	___	___
Do you eat until your stomach hurts?	___	___
Does eating cause you to fall asleep?	___	___
Do certain occasions require certain foods?	___	___
In your lifetime have you lost more than 50 pounds?	___	___
Does a "good" restaurant serve large portions?	___	___
Do you eat snacks before going out to eat with others?	___	___
Do you eat standing up?	___	___
Do you inhale your food?	___	___
Do you become irritated at postponed eating?	___	___
Have you heard others call food "too rich" and felt confused?	___	___

	YES	NO
Do you awake from sleep to eat?	___	___
Does your wardrobe vary three sizes or more?	___	___
Does eating sometimes make you hungrier than not eating?	___	___
Do you feel like an object as others describe your body?	___	___
Have you felt people should, "love me, love my fat"?	___	___
Do you usually clean your plate whether hungry or not?	___	___
Is your eating rather continuous?	___	___
At a party, do you spend most of your time at the snack table, or do you consciously avoid the food area?	___	___
Have you tried more than one fad diet?	___	___
Do you make fun of yourself before others can?	___	___
Do you feel exhilarated when you control food?	___	___
Are you afraid to be "normal"?	___	___
When you know certain foods are on the shelf do they "call" to you?	___	___
Do you buy clothes either too big or too small?	___	___
Do your friends eat like you do and are they embarrassed?	___	___
Do you postpone joys with "wait 'til I control my weight"?	___	___
Do others see your shape differently than you do?	___	___

Chapter Two

Who's an E-D?

Who's an E-D? Maybe you are! By picking up this book, you've shown some interest in eating disorders, fat, health, dieting, etc. Many people, in order to live as full-blooded, card-carrying Americans, need some kind of substance abuse to cope. There are 60–80 million fat Americans, 30 percent of all college women binge and vomit, and one in ten high school girls are anorexic. It seems America's "drug of choice" is food. If you use food to cope with life rather than to stoke your engines, you are an E-D. This applies whether your unnatural relationship is one of bingeing excessive quantities, or swearing off into starvation. These are merely opposite sides of the same coin. E-Ds eat or starve in order to cope and compete.

IT'S HARD AS HELL!

Suffering an eating disorder is woven into every cell of your being and cannot be exorcised with a quickie diet or brief stint in psychotherapy. It's really bigger than all that. If those simple solutions would have worked, you would not be looking at this book.

Paying attention to the seriousness and difficulty of this is not meant to depress you. Instead, it is meant to comfort and encourage. You have spent much of your life hearing how easy this project of control of food should be. That made you feel much worse. After all, you failed at such an easy task. Instead, let's say that this recovery from your eating disorder will be *the hardest thing you've ever undertaken.* Everything else you've done was accomplished with your best friend, food. This project, you'll take on without the comfort of food.

It seems so much more honest and humane to warn you in advance and let you know that we know how hard it is rather than all that stiff upper lip minimizing. I found this true in my life when I underwent a minor surgical procedure. The doctor told me I would feel pain for a few minutes. I decided that meant three minutes. For me, *a couple* would be two minutes and *a few* meant three. As it turned out, I remained in pain for twenty minutes until the anesthetic took effect. Later I told the doctor I was concerned that maybe I had complications because I hurt for so long. He quickly brushed my concerns aside as he assured me that most people hurt for about twenty minutes. In his vocabulary, *a few* meant twenty minutes! I remarked to him that I might have been less fearful and agitated if I had known exactly how many minutes I would hurt. In other words, I might have been more willing to flow with the pain and cooperate with my body. As it was, I became fearful, expecting the pain to end much sooner than predicted. I would have preferred some clearer advance warning about what was ahead. When I told the doctor about my experience, he cautioned that if he told people to expect pain, they might "manufacture" more than necessary. There are advantages and disadvantages either way.

I have found it is better to let E-Ds know in advance how painful recovery will be. Too much time and money has been spent on minimizing, pretending, and hoping for easier ways. You will now look at the seriousness as a way to face the problem. After you acknowledge it will be hard, you will be shown a way out.

MOVING FROM SIN TO SICKNESS

How many times have you said, "I was really 'bad' during the holidays, but I'm going to be 'good' for the new year"? You have been using food as a way to evaluate "good" and "bad." In actuality, your eating behavior has nothing at all to do with whether you are a sinner or a saint. You have an illness. You have tried your best to control your compulsive relationship with food, but all to no avail. Finally, medical science is catching up to this reality. There are now clinical diagnoses for people who suffer from eating disorders.

You are not a bad person, but a sick person. It was not until 1957 that the American Medical Association declared alcoholism a disease. For centuries before that, alcoholics died from their compulsion to drink. Similarly, schizophrenics were jailed and tortured before investigation revealed their underlying chemical and psychological malady.

My major motivation in creating hospital eating disorder units was so the patient could move from the sin to sickness model. I had seen that such an approach had done wonders for alcoholics. Receiving treatment in a hospital setting, where a doctor acknowledged the seriousness of the illness and the patient got respect rather than punishment, helped the patient become willing to get well. Eating disorder sufferers need the same respect and attention to their serious, lifelong, chronic illness. The minimizing, punitive solutions haven't worked. Let's take a serious look at your illness.

If you have chosen food as your drug of choice, you clinically fall into one of two major categories of eating disorders: bulimia or anorexia. In this book, I combine these two disorders because, in my experience, they are really the same illness. Psychologically, both exhibit the same personality profiles. To divide you into categories, fat or thin, is unrealistic. You both have the same personality structures and therefore need the same treatment in order to recover. One of you is fat, the other thin. In fact, some may even be both—a person whose weight changes frequently, never maintaining a stable body configuration. Quite possibly, you weighed 90 pounds last year and ate only lettuce, but this year you weigh 180 pounds and can't stand to be around "normal" friends. You can't stand people who like anything other than going out to dinner. Very often an E-D's body changes as frequently as the weather. As a patient once quipped to me, "I was thin once—during a half-hour flight over Chicago."

More than likely you have experienced both slim and chunky bodies. Some with childhood onset obesity have special metabolic, genetic, and cultural problems, but even those have also had periods of slimness. (Even if only during airline flights!) In nearly all cases, anorexics started out with overweight problems, began dieting, got high off not eating, and now are emaciated and obsessed with avoiding food. Still, food remains the number one topic in life.

Whether fat or thin, you really contain the ingredient of your opposite side. If thin, you are surely repulsed by the fat lady and don't want her anywhere around. Fat ladies say, "What do I have in common with a skinny little bitch like that? She flaunts her body!" In either case, your recovery will depend on making friends with that opposite side of yourself you'd rather avoid. Your biggest project at hand right now will be to remove poundage as your criteria of evaluation, whether of yourself or others. You will have to see that the disorder is in your relationship with food, not your poundage.

Recovery will involve renegotiating your relationship with food, not obsessing about the poundage on your scale.

FORSAKE THE SCALE GOD

If you have bought what I propose thus far you can surely see the absurdity in going to your health spa and bragging to your friends that, "I just lost three pounds!" That's the same three or thirty pounds you lost last year and the year before. Poundage is not the issue! You must be ready to have a totally new relationship with food. Bowing down to a scale every morning is all part of the obsession. That very behavior must stop.

You have made the scale your god. Each morning you bow down to ask, "Who am I, God?" You are really asking this god, "Did I get away with it?" You want to know if there were any consequences to the eating you already feel guilty about. If you ate and didn't gain, you sigh, "Phew, I got away with it." Maybe you check in with the scale god because you are dieting and you want quick reinforcement for your deprivation. You bow down to ask the god, "Do I get a quick payoff for my suffering?" In either case, you are looking to an external, spring-driven contraption to verify who you are. Whether the scale god shows a loss or a gain, it is usually an excuse to binge. If you've lost weight, you say, "Well, I'm doing pretty well, no need to rush it, I think I'll eat a little." If you haven't lost weight, you complain, "This isn't fair, I may as well eat." In either case, weighing leads to eating. Weigh yourself right now, as you begin this book, and then don't weigh again for one month. You may find that it is harder to give up the scale than to give up the food. Try it and see what happens.

As you give up the focus on poundage, you become more ready to accept your illness as a medical reality instead of a moral affliction. Let's take a look at the diagnostic categories.

BULIMIA

"Bulimia" is derived from the Greek work *buli* which means "to eat like an animal, or animal hunger." It does not mean "vomiting," even though that has evolved in popular usage. If you are to be medically diagnosed as having bulimia, your doctor will ask certain questions about your relationship with food.

The following questions are derived from the diagnostic category of bulimia, and you can use them to see if you fit the category. Answer as truthfully as possible, even though some parts of your relationship with food will be a secret even to you.

1. Do you binge (take in large amounts of food in brief periods of time)?
2. Are you aware that your eating pattern is abnormal?
3. Do you feel depressed and put yourself down after a binge?
4. Do you feel that, once you start a binge, you can't stop yourself voluntarily? (Are you out of control with your food?)

In the following questions, a "yes" answer to *any three* means you can be diagnosed as bulimic.

5. When you binge, do you eat high calorie foods that you can take in easily?
6. When you binge, is it often in secret and hidden?
7. To stop bingeing, do you vomit, fall asleep, wait until someone interrupts you, or cringe in pain? (In other words, is it rarely a clear decision to stop eating?)
8. Do you often have weight fluctuations of ten pounds or more?
9. Have you repeatedly tried to lose weight by restrictive diets, vomiting, laxatives, diuretics, or medications to make you vomit?

These are the kinds of questions a doctor would ask. As you can see, only one question pertains to weight and it refers only to the speed with which you put it on and take it off. Bulimia has nothing to do with weight. You can be fat and a binger, or you can be thin and a binger. The illness is the unnatural manner of "shoveling in" food. Also notice that some questions pertain to vomiting, but you do not have to vomit to be bulimic. Bingeing and then dieting restrictively is a form of bulimia. You may secretly binge on corn chips, fall asleep, and then wake up depressed and ten pounds heavier. Your solution might be to fast and guzzle laxatives until the weight disappears. This is bulimia.

Bulimia refers to the manner in which you take in food, not how it gets out. You may keep the binge in, as fat, or you may vomit it out, or diet it off. The main ingredient of bulimia is bingeing.

Popularized in television newscasts and recent magazine exposes, the term *bulimarexia* has come into our vocabulary to designate people who binge and then vomit. This term is not in professional writings, but is used by the public. If you binge and then vomit, you can rest assured that just simple "bulimia" is what you've got.

ANOREXIA

Now, what if you are just as obsessed with food, but to the opposite extreme? You are driven and obsessed *not* to eat. The following are questions a doctor would ask in diagnosing you as anorexic. Try to answer these for yourself as honestly as you can. A major problem in trying to diagnose yourself is your own denial. You may not see the situation clearly. If you are anorexic, other people in your life may point this out long before you recognize the problem.

1. Do you have an intense fear of becoming obese?
2. Even if you are successful on a weight loss program, do you still maintain an intense fear of obesity?
3. Do you feel fat even when others tell you you are emaciated?
4. Have you lost at least 25 percent of your minimal body weight as projected for your age and height?
5. Do you adamantly refuse to maintain the average body weight medically recommended for you?
6. Have you felt excessive coldness, swelling, low blood pressure, and slow pulse?
7. If female, do you menstruate irregularly or not at all?
8. Do you sometimes eat and then vomit?

In anorexia as well as bulimia, it is not your weight that is of utmost importance. The essential factor is your attitude toward food and dieting. If anorexic, you have an unnatural fear of food. You may be repulsed by your own body, especially if it is normal. The third question, referring to a distorted image of your own body's appearance, is crucial to both anorexia and bulimia. Fat people see themselves as thinner than they really are, and skinny people feel fat. You can see, therefore, how these disorders come from internal messages and have nothing to do with weight. They have more to do with accepting reality and yourself. Ultimately, the recovery program for both eating disorders must include finding a way to love yourself and get more love from others. That is why "fat is a family affair."

YOU ARE AN ADDICT!

Although the recovery from eating disorders is psychological and emotional, we cannot underestimate the physical component to these illnesses. I have grave concerns about the direction of medical science, diagnosing these illnesses as purely psychological. This is exactly what was done with alcoholics years ago as they were put into mental hospitals rather than alcoholism treatment centers. Professionals denied that some of the abnormal behavior was a result of drinking. With E-Ds, some abnormality is caused by the eating. After alcoholism treatment units showed patients with successful recoveries, we found that only two percent really had any serious psychological illness which required treatment. That is the same proportion as the general population.

Treatment for addictive disorders follows a different approach than treatment for psychiatric disorders. If the psychiatric approach might have worked, I surely would not have attained 222 pounds!

There is a strong physical component to eating disorders. My own lifelong effort to avoid that issue kept me in extensive insight therapy for ten years laboring to find out why I ate. I presumed that when I figured out why, I would miraculously stop eating. Unfortunately, therapy helped me deny there was a physical component to my illness. If I did not stop overeating first, I would not be awake enough to honestly examine why. In other words, food is a drug. Excess food dulls the senses and relieves pain. It takes the edge off. It works!

Every addict, no matter what the substance, has to learn one day that the relationship is harmful. By picking up this book you acknowledge that you may have a destructive relationship with food. This admission is at least embarrassing and perhaps disconcerting. It is not glamorous to acknowledge that a piece of chocolate cake has got the better of you. I often wished I were an alcoholic instead of a compulsive overeater. Alcoholics include famous jazz musicians, senators, comic and serious movie stars, even space heroes. Who of note ever admitted to needing to eat, no matter what price, and to having an unnatural, destructive response to a Twinkie? This is the E-D's dilemma. Perhaps thirty years ago, when the first alcoholics were coming out of the closets, they had similar trauma.

WHAT IS AN ADDICT?

A simple, but workable definition of addiction is, "When you don't have it, you feel bad; when you have it, you don't feel good." This may be where you find yourself in your relationship with food. Despite the way it seems to smooth out the rough edges, it doesn't help you really soar with your life. You don't wake up joyous and happy to be alive. In fact, in the latter stages of addiction, you may wake up slightly hung over from the binge of the night before. You will overeat because you have to, not because you want to. By the time you recognize that this substance has the best of you, you are well into full-blown addiction. Medical science characterized three distinct aspects of addiction which apply to those addicted to food:

1) There is initially a *high tolerance* for the substance.

This is apparent when you find yourself eating everyone out of the house and home. You can put away much larger quantities than others, and then experience minimal, if any, discomfort. You may also find others commenting that some foods are "too rich." You are puzzled by what "rich" means. As they push away these rich plates, you finish them up while clearing the table. Your tolerance for the substance is quite different from others.

2) *Withdrawals* when removed.

If you have found yourself sluggish and irritable when trying to diet, you are experiencing light withdrawal symptoms. Some E-Ds experience anything from violent tremors, inappropriate mood swings, crying, shaking, and sometimes even convulsing. Medical science has not adequately monitored these withdrawal symptoms, as we have just begun to establish hospital units with this specialty. In the early days of alcoholism treatment, sufferers complained of withdrawal symptoms and medical personnel tended to minimize these reports. Possibly, some of this medical minimizing was due to the physician's own drinking pattern. "Everyone likes to have a drink once in a while." Even medical personnel don't want to acknowledge the dire consequences when drinking is carried to excess. We are quite willing to acknowledge the monstrous effects of heroin withdrawal. A little-known fact is that people can die in the throes of alcohol withdrawal, but rarely die in heroin withdrawal. It hurts, but it doesn't kill. Alcohol, like food, bathes every single body cell, and therefore it affects every single organ system. If we minimized alcohol's addictive qualities because we all wanted to drink, imagine what kind of minimizing and denial goes on with food withdrawals.

The following are some symptoms of sugar withdrawal:

fatigue	crying spells
dizziness	poor memory
irritability	mood swings
depression	temper outbursts
fainting spells	blurred vision
insomnia	indigestion
night sweats	asthma
suicidal tendencies	impotence
shaking	headaches

The worst withdrawals occur in the fourth through the sixth day of recovery. If you can let yourself sit and shake and cry or whatever you have to do, the discomfort will pass. Unfortunately, rarely has anyone addressed how hard it will be, so when you felt these withdrawals before, you just self-medicated yourself with more food. If you have trouble accepting this addiction idea, just consider how many times you've given up your "diet" on Thursdays (the fourth day). You always start on a Monday, and when Thursday's withdrawals start, you decide instead to binge for the weekend and "start fresh next week."

3) *Cravings* after withdrawal.

Even after you have given up the offending substance, you will still experience psychological cravings long after the physical pangs have ended. These cravings are what takes every sufferer back to the offending substance. You miss what the old standby did for your feelings. When the feelings become too much to handle, when life intrudes on diet plans, it seems simpler to return to the substance than to change your life. With the plan outlined in this book you will find a way to diminish the cravings because you are going to change your life.

ADDICTED TO WHAT?

If you have been raised on a typical American diet off supermarket shelves, more than likely you are a "junk food junkie." Your addiction is to simple sugars and refined carbohydrates. Eating too much of anything will put excess sugar into your system. There are numerous nutrition treatises which will explain this in greater detail. Though you didn't ask to be an addict, it seems you've ended up here. When I worked with heroin addicts on the streets of New York, their evolution to addiction differed greatly from the gradual and insidious addiction of alcoholics and E-Ds. Heroin abusers knew they were injecting an illegal substance and they knew it was addictive. They made a conscious decision to become addicts and accept the consequences. You, unfortunately, are finding yourself addicted without asking for it and certainly never intending to end up here. What happened?

Some explanation comes from the works of Manuel Cheraskin, nutritionist, dentist, and researcher at Louisiana State University. In his book, *Psychodietetics,* Dr. Cheraskin told of feeding a group of mice delicious mouse food pellets full of nutrients and fiber, and low in salt, sugar, and fat. He gave these mice a choice of drinking water or alcohol. They were all repulsed by the alcohol and chose water. Later he separated the mice and kept half of the group on mouse pellets while the other half were fed junk foods from Cheetos to Fritos; salami to chocolate cake. The second groups of mice, when offered a beverage, chose alcohol instead of water. What does this mean? These junk food mice were experiencing "withdrawals" from the sugars and alcohol soothed the raw edges. (Alcohol is sugar in liquid form.) The mice, like humans, needed soothing when coming off junk foods. Are we raising a nation of alcoholics as well?

These questions have also been pondered by William Dufty in *Sugar Blues,* where he makes a case for sugar addiction. American consumption of sugar has grown to 125 pounds per person per year! Hidden sugar is found in nearly every packaged product on the grocer's shelf. Even baby food is loaded with sugar, not for the baby, but because the mother prefers the taste. Long before the poor baby can decide, it is addicted and withdrawing. Even cigarette tobacco is laced with sugar in the curing process. It is interesting to note how many people who give up smoking cigarettes turn to eating sugar compulsively. Alcoholics crave sugar when giving up booze. Without the personality change, we may all simply transfer addictions and stay in the cycle.

SAYS WHO?

Are you aggravated? I don't blame you. After all, who wants to think of themselves as an addict? "I can handle this whenever I want to" is the woeful refrain of every addict. "I just don't want to yet." When you sit down honestly and alone with this book, you must ultimately acknowledge what you have always known to be true. It does have the best of you, maybe not forever, but at least for today. The idea of sugar as an addiction is quite controversial. Physicians who read this book will probably write angry letters about the use of an addictive model with eating disorders. I once gave a presentation to a group of prominent doctors. Among the group was a short man who angrily denounced what I was saying. He claimed the sugar addiction idea was a fallacy. "There is no scientific evidence to prove what you are purporting here!" he shouted. "I have been an endocrinologist for many years and have found no scientific evidence to corroborate these ideas." I offer you the same answer I offered him. "Even though this may not as yet be proved, it helps people get off their own backs and gets them out of a punitive, self-loathing cycle. They can then see themselves as sick people seeking a cure rather than degenerates wanting pity. The addictive model takes morality out of eating disorders."

Maybe medical science hasn't yet caught up with what you already know about your eating behavior. You know it's an addiction. Your recovery will be similar to what works for other addicts.

BUT I'M ANOREXIC AND DON'T EAT AT ALL!

Even if your refusal of food keeps you suffering, the addiction model still applies. As an anorexic, you are addicted to the high, clean, superhuman feeling you have when you don't eat. There is a physical high that comes from not eating. Hindu mystics have encouraged fasting for centuries as a way to seek enlightenment, spiritual fulfillment, and lightheaded ecstacy. You may crave that clean feeling and feel sluggish, repulsive withdrawals when you try to eat. Early in 1983, the New England Journal of Medicine published a highly controversial study which compared feelings and lifestyles of anorexic teenage girls and 40-year-old male runners. They both felt exhilarated by the feeling of pushing their bodies past the normal limits of human endurance. Runners call this "hitting the wall." Anorexics often delight in testing their endurance. They serve elaborate meals to others and eat nothing themselves. It is the same type of high. Many anorexics have a drugged look; they stare blankly as if not involved in what is going on around them. Runners report the same "alone" trancelike state when they exhaust themselves. Their "runner's high" is just as addicting as the anorexic's starvation.

GIMME FUZZIES

William Glasser, M.D., in his book, *Positive Addiction,* outlines some of these tendencies toward psychological dependency. There is more research now underway which shows strong evidence of an actual *physical* component to these addictions. In the early 1970s, doctors began studying a mechanism within the nervous system which produces a morphine-like effect helping to alleviate pain and subduing trauma and shock.

These morphine-like substances are called *endorphins* and they are secreted to soothe pain, take the edge off, and promote general well-being. Some research indicates that overeaters and alcoholics produce fewer of these endorphins than normal people. Medical science is currently researching evidence that some metabolisms break down sugar differently than others. Sugar works to soothe the savage beast. Since you produce fewer endorphins, you often feel on a raw edge. Eating sugar increases endorphin production, so when you eat, the rawness vanishes. Some people don't get the same effects from sugar. That is the reason they can take it or leave it. They are already soothed by the endorphins they produce naturally.

If anorexic, you get the same kind of soothing from the "high" of not eating. That exuberant feeling comes from the endurance high of pushing yourself beyond your limits, much like the "runner's high" mentioned earlier. These sedating feelings are hard to give up. But don't despair, there is an alternative method to increase endorphin production and it doesn't involve bingeing or deprivation. It involves hugging. That's right, hugging. When you turn to a fellow human being and you put your arms around one another, this starts the endorphins flowing and the raw edges are removed by the warmth of a loving friend. Your dog is no dummy when he jumps up for a rub on the chest or pat on the head. He's getting his endorphins up and keeping himself mellow.

Animals in nature huddle and cuddle whenever they want to. How many obesity treatment programs are begun to treat animals? They get their hugs and don't need to binge. The only overweight animals are those force-fed by humans, or domestic pets of people who, fat themselves, overfeed to show love.

The Chinese are high on hugs and low on obesity. In China, mothers carry babies on their backs or slung at their sides for many years. The baby is rarely far from the warmth of the mother's body, and, when hungry, is brought immediately to the breast. They also deal with discipline differently than in the U.S. Babies are not disciplined until age five, when they are considered at the "age of reason" and thus able to distinguish right from wrong. Despite the few exceptions who gain weight to show wealth, the Chinese do not have obesity problems. To give up food you need to take in love. If you find this idea embarrassing, do it for health reasons. Hug medicinally. You have to get hugs to keep from eating. It's all part of your recovery.

"WILLPOWER" DIED OF OBESITY

Other people who don't suffer as you do will sometimes try to tell you it's all in your mind. This is a variation on the "use a little willpower" approach. Even though you do suffer physical withdrawal and can see the strong addictive aspect to having an eating disorder, there is also the influence of the mind addiction. It has to do with your attitude when you take in food—your relationship with food. A normal person seeks food to alleviate hunger or provide sustenance and does not worry about being "bad." The most predominant attitude toward eating suffered by the obese as well as the anorexic is guilt. When eating is accompanied by guilt, you're in trouble. Normal people don't eat with guilt. If they are going to be guilty, they simply refrain. E-Ds project the guilt, wallow in it, beat themselves for it, and then eat anyway!

When the American Medical Association initially declared alcoholism a disease, one element in diagnosing the illness was looking for "A PERSON WHO HAS *TRIED* TO QUIT." If the person had tried to stop the behavior and still kept it up, it was an indication they were addicted. You see, normal people don't *try* to quit. If they see a problem with certain behavior, they just stop it. If they don't see a problem, they have no need to even think about quitting. An addict *tries* to quit. Over and over and over again, an addict tries to control an obsessive relationship with food, and, despite brief periods of control, returns to obsessive addiction.

You've tried to quit and couldn't. You judged yourself harshly instead of accepting that you suffer from an illness and can't help it. More than likely, you eat compulsively with an inordinate amount of both guilt and despair. Remember, in diagnosing bulimia and anorexia, doctors look for the attitude a patient has toward eating. Let's look at attitude as it related to alcoholism, and see if you can draw any parallels to your own addiction. When drinking is done with guilt, the incidence of alcoholism is much greater. This is clear in Mormon and Moslem populations. Both groups look upon drinking alcohol as sinful. When a person from either of these groups drinks even a slight amount of alcohol, guilt and remorse immediately set in. They often drink to cover the guilt, and they end up drunk nearly every time. I found clients from both of these groups the hardest to treat. These clients found great difficulty in moving from the sin to the sickness model. In order to recover, you must accept that you are ill. When the power of food to make you "good" or "bad" is removed, you will stop turning to willpower and ask instead for help from other people.

YOUR ILLNESS IS A DISEASE

You have a *dis*ease when you are not at "ease." Something is wrong. Alcoholism is a disease and so are eating disorders. When we think of this disease, we divide it into a *physical addiction* coupled with a *psychological obsession*. We just discussed some of the physiology. Nearly all your efforts at controlling the disease have centered around physical approaches, not on the addictive quality of eating.

Some have even cut out half their intestines to gain control of the eating. Even after drastic surgeries, many regained lost weight. Without treatment of the psychological aspects, the organism will not change. You must acknowledge the physical aspects, but also look at the psychological obsession. You can't minimize either part of the disease. Let's take a look at the gradual and insidious progression of the psychological aspects of this obsession.

EAT TO CELEBRATE AND EAT TO MOURN

A full-fledged E-D eats in any heightened awareness state. You eat to level out emotions, good or bad. You eat to achieve numbness. You eat when your team wins and you eat when it loses. It is pointless to ponder the reasons for eating. Such investigations may prove interesting to you after you have stopped the eating, but for now, they accomplish little. As long as eating helps you sedate and soothes the rough edges, you won't really uncover true and clear information to help you. Therapy for someone who is still eating compulsively is like talking with someone who is drunk. Insight does not change eating behavior. Changing eating behavior however, can change insight. You got this far, slowly and insidiously, over a long period of time. It is practically impossible to be aware of this gradual progression while you are in it.

PROGRESSION TOWARD PSYCHOLOGICAL OBSESSION

Check if you:

WARNING SIGNALS
_____ Have a hereditary propensity for overeating
_____ Have a low tolerance for "negative" feelings (anger, sadness, fear, etc.)
_____ Have a high stress level
_____ Resent thin or normal people and often feel in competition with them

ABUSE
_____ Use food to escape worries
_____ Use food to hide from other issues (sexual, employment, etc.)

_____ Spend too much time thinking about food (shopping, cooking, dining out)

_____ Avoid discussions about food and weight, or constantly discuss food and weight

_____ "Diet" constantly (fasting, bingeing, bulimia)

_____ Secretly eat in public (while shopping or driving)

_____ Anticipate shortages and overeat to avoid "hunger"

_____ Feel compelled to eat again and again within a short period of time or soon after a meal

ADDICTION

_____ Eat to the point of bloating or nausea

_____ Eat to relieve negative feelings (guilt, shame, remorse) from overeating

_____ Deny weight gain, or see no relation between food eaten and weight gained

_____ Deny physical damage and/or complications

_____ Deny powerlessness, make promises to limit or control eating and then break these promises again and again

_____ Have periods of memory loss (blackouts), go into a trance-like state while eating

_____ Lack awareness of quantities in normal portions

_____ Feel trapped (food is salvation as well as destruction)

_____ Make desperate attempts to control eating and weight through fad diets, pills, sweat suits, exercise classes, etc.

_____ Frequently feel shame, guilt, remorse after failure and eat for relief

_____ Lie about eating or other behaviors; steal food or money for food

_____ Feel scared or "different"—alienated from other people

_____ Find your eating interferes with normal activities or relationships (job, family, community)

_____ Feel hopeless, anxious, depressed, or suicidal

EARLY STAGES

If you were born to two fat parents, you have an 80 percent chance of being fat yourself. You have a genetic tendency to accumulate fat cells. From the starting gate, you already have a few strikes against you. Now, do you think fat parents will be teaching you to eat normally? Most likely, not. You will be trained early to overeat. You will learn that, what others might call "humongous" portions, your family sees as meager. You will develop a style of overeating. Both heredity and environment play a part in determining your future as an E-D. Most important, however, is your training to use food to relieve stress. In a stressful environment, you are programmed to take that rough edge off through the use of a simple, time-honored, immediate ritual—put something in your mouth. You don't know any other way to reduce stress. You don't consider that changing your life could help reduce stress. Food is immediate and easy. You develop a style of expecting immediate relief or immediate gratification. You do not practice deferring gratification. ("I want what I want when I want it!") You learned this attitude long before the "age of reason," and it will be hard to give up even after the "dawn of insight." Because you didn't practice deferring, you have a very low tolerance to stress. You don't know how to weather it; you only know how to smother it. So, as you grow and your life becomes even more complicated, you have more stresses and more need for food. The needs increase without your own awareness.

OBSESSIONAL STAGE

Since you have fashioned a lifestyle with food abuse at its base, you will have to carefully guard both your supplies and your consumption. A slight embarrassment may be creeping in about the amounts you eat and how you "shovel," so you may start to take more meals and snacks alone. Sometimes these times will be stolen moments away from a crowd and you will have to gulp your food quickly so no one will find you out. This gives rise to a pattern of eating even if you don't feel like it. You will be eating out of fear—the fear that you may end up hungry. You don't want to be out socially and appear hungry. You don't want people to think you overeat. So, to forestall any problem, you eat at home to "get a buzz on" before the party to help you endure the difficulty of making small talk. You don't enjoy or savor your eating, but instead eat "just in case." You become preoccupied with food and shopping and insuring that you will get "enough." By this time, however, enough is never enough.

SECRET LIFE

You know you are out of control. Brief moments of clarity arise, but you quickly eat to avoid them. Food makes you feel better and takes away the guilt momentarily. Guilty about your eating behavior, you eat to make that feeling go away. You develop a denial system to convince yourself "it's not that bad." Your eating becomes a secret, not only to others, but also to yourself. You eat while shopping or standing over a sink. You deny all weight gains. You see no relationship between the food in your mouth and the fat on your body. At the time you are eating, you completely block out the possibility of consequences. You have been learning how to fast and then binge, so in the moment of eating, you tell yourself, "It doesn't count. I'll fast tomorrow." This develops the "catch-up" phenomenon. Binge today, fast tomorrow. The pendulum swings from excess and numbness to guilt and "swearing off." Eventually you learn how to turn off even this denial mechanism. You resent thin or normal people and avoid discussions of food or dieting. "If I ignore it," you hope, "it will go away."

FULL-FLEDGED COMPULSION

Instead of going away, it gets worse. You continue eating until nauseated, even though food no longer works. You feel unable to cope emotionally, and to complicate things, you start having physical withdrawals periodically as you make futile attempts at testing your willpower. Even though food does not work, you have no other tools for coping, so you keep on the same merry-go-round, returning to food again and again. Sometimes you even experience periods of memory loss as you become excessively preoccupied with food and weight. Nothing else matters. "When I get thin" it will all matter again. With no memory, you can conveniently forget the quantities you are eating. When moments of clarity do arise, you resort to elaborate alibis and justifications for your eating. Since you can't truly believe you are out of control, you project reasons for this weird behavior "out there." It is hard to believe that your best friend, food, has turned on you; that despite what you eat, you still feel moody, depressed, and grouchy. It must be *them*: "Who wouldn't eat with a life like mine? My stressful job and boss force me to binge."

GETTING READY

At some point, the alibi system will break down and you become ready to change your life and give up the obsession. Dishonesty about your food intake has spread to dishonesty in your whole life. You deny to yourself that "This is my life." Instead, you see life as a dress rehearsal. Life will begin "when I get thin." You lose self-esteem by continually breaking promises to yourself. You begin grandiose, perfectionistic behavior as a coverup. You may resort to a PIP (Privileged Invalid Position) to complain to everyone that you "can't help it." As badly as you feel, you keep drawing attention to yourself. Your entire identity revolves around being a person with a weight problem. You are trying to get out of the problem, but don't know how. With repeated failure, you return yet again to food. However, what used to solve problems now becomes a problem in itself. With any luck, you come to see that you have to stop the yo-yo cycle with food. Then you can see what your life is really about. You can only be ready when you are ready. At this ready stage you are not only fed up with food and its effects, but you are *sick and tired of being sick and tired.*

Chapter Three

Who's a Codependent?

A codependent under/overeater is someone whose life is intertwined with the person who has an eating disorder. Their mission in life is to *cure* the food abuse. They forget their own lives to help another's. The codependent has often been overlooked in eating disorder rehabilitation. Actually, they are a partner in keeping the food abuse continuing. In the early '60s when alcoholism treatment programs were beginning to take form, no one paid attention to family members. It was assumed that these people had no specific needs. We also assumed they would be ecstatic when their alcoholic stopped drinking. We found instead that when a spouse's drinking stopped, depression sometimes emerged in the partner. Some family members actually worked to sabotage the alcoholic's treatment! They needed the alcoholic's return to drinking. If, by chance, the alcoholic's recovery was not sabotaged, many formerly "helpful" spouses sought divorce instead. They had stayed during all the bad times, but when change came, they had to leave. Often they left to marry another alcoholic. I once treated a woman who had married several alcoholics, one of them twice. She adamantly swore off with each divorce, but without examining her own needs and wants as a codependent personality, she was doomed to repeat her endless cycle.

An addict in recovery from an eating disorder presents difficulty and necessary change for the codependent. In this book codependents will find help to survive recovery.

We're *all* codependent. That's right. We are all people whose lives have been affected by someone else's eating disorder. We care. We want to help. And, most importantly, we feel frustrated by not knowing what to do. To specifically diagnose a codependent, we need to see exactly how much one person's life is intertwined with the other's.

CONFLUENCE

In describing a *confluent* personality type, we refer to people who have no sense of their own ego boundaries. In other words, it is hard for them to know where they stop and another person begins. Everyone seems to ebb and flow into each other. "When you have a splinter, my finger hurts." This quality of being perceptive and aware of the other person, the ability to walk in another's shoes, is often an asset. Such confluence makes many terrific actors and actresses, nurses, doctors, and psychologists. As a codependent, your confluence also helps in dangerous situations, as you develop a healthy caution. You can deftly sense what is going on in the other person. In families, however, this confluence leads into a tangled web where you lose your own identity in the service of others. In addictive families, members become so enmeshed in each other's needs and identities that it takes extensive work to get untangled. Each family member will have to learn how to speak for him- or herself and develop separateness. You may think you know what your loved one is thinking long before they say it. Often you may be right, but assuming you've got them figured out is actually disrespectful. You rob them of the chance to feel like an exciting, evolving person around you. You also rob yourself of the chance to be surprised and learn something new about your relationship. Recovery is a whole new ball game.

It is safe to say that a codependent is *someone who is addicted to another's addiction.* Codependents take on curing the E-D as their mission in life. They become obsessed with solving their loved ones' problems. Whether their E-D is fat or emaciated, the codependent takes on the role of food monitor and diet prescriber. On the one hand, codependents relish the idea of discussing their E-D's problems, yet often have great difficulty talking about their own lives. (It is important to note that an E-D can also be a codependent.) Many fat people keep others who are even fatter around so they can worry about them instead of themselves. It could even become a "mutual suicide pact" where an alcoholic and an overeater are involved: "I won't say anything about your drinking if you won't say anything about my eating." A codependent's involvement in the E-D's problems extends beyond caring to a dogged insistence on being able to solve the problem. Anorexic girls often control their mothers by alternately demanding and rejecting help. The codependent starts to suffer as much or more than the E-D. This is especially true in anorexia, where we see fearful and distraught parents whose daughters shrug and sneer, "no problem." Real compassion is helping others solve a problem, not feeling it more than they do.

You may be reading this book because of your emotional involvement with someone who is suffering from one of the eating disorders. More than likely, you're also hurting. You are strongly invested in helping this person. You may even be more involved and interested in that person's life than he or she seems to be. You are the one providing the energy and impetus to the relationship while your E-D is *out to lunch!* This chapter is for you. The following attitudes are signs of impending codependency.

"I feel safest when I am giving."
"I know more clearly what you want than what I want."
"I only feel good about myself if I have your approval."
"I am very concerned with how you look because you are a reflection of me."
"When you are hurting, I often feel it more deeply than you do."
"If you have a bad day, I react."
"If you have problems, I feel I must come up with a solution for you."
"I need to be needed."
"I don't develop many of my own interests, but respond to yours."
"Before speaking, I carefully gauge what effect and reaction I want to achieve from you."
"If someone is angry with me, I find that intolerable."
"I diminish my social circle to get overly involved in you."
"I focus on your problems a lot so I won't have to face any of my own."
"I am critical and judgmental, then I feel guilty."
"I think I can convince you to like yourself."

Codependents need help as much as the person with the eating disorder. They need help to take care of themselves without guilt or excessive feelings of responsibility. Whenever I lecture on the family aspect of overeating, most participants expect three fairly standard discussions. They think I want to talk about 1) the *genetic* aspects of obesity, 2) how families need to adjust to *new food plans,* or 3) how family members can best *help* their loved one maintain their commitment to a food plan. I address none of those topics. For help with food, I recommend professional nutritionists, or others similarly afflicted, like people in Overeaters Anonymous. As to the food plan, that's not the family's business. Regarding genetics, at this point, it doesn't make much difference how we got here. We all need help getting out. The discussion must instead center on codependents getting help in order to detach with love.

ARE YOU A CODEPENDENT?

Use this questionnaire to evaluate the extent of your involvement.

Do you force diets?

Do you threaten to leave due to weight?

Do you check on the diet?

Do you make promises based on pounds lost or gained?

Do you hide food from an overeater?

Do you worry incessantly about an undereater?

Have you "walked on eggshells" so as not to upset the over/under-
eater?

Do you throw food away so the overeater won't find it?

Have you excused the erratic, sometimes violent, mood swings result-
ing from sugar binges?

Do you change social activities so the overeater won't be tempted?

Do you manipulate budgets to control spending on food and clothing?

Do you purchase and promote eating the "right" foods?

Do you promote gyms, health spas, and miracle cures?

Do you break into emotional tirades when you catch the overeater
bingeing?

Are you constantly disappointed when you see relapse?

Are you embarrassed by over/undereater's appearance?

Do you falsely console the over/undereater when they are embarrassed?

Do you set up tests of willpower to tease the over/undereater?
Have you lowered your expectations of what you might like?
Does your weight fluctuate with your loved one's (you up, they down)?
Have you stopped attending to your own grooming?
Do you have many aches and pains, and preoccupation with health?
Are you drinking heavily or using sleeping pills or tranquilizers?
Do you bribe with food?
Do you talk about the eater's body to them or others?
Do you feel life will be perfect if they shape up?
Are you grateful you aren't "that bad"?
Does their eating disorder give you license to run away?
Does their eating disorder give you an excuse to stay?
Do you "subtly" leave "helpful" literature around the house?
Do you read diet books though you have no weight problem?
Do you think you have the perfect home, except for the E-D?
Do you use pills to get to sleep and escape worry?
Have you spent much time in your own therapy talking about the E-D?

If you found the foregoing guide descriptive of your relationship, read on! This book will show you the benefits to be gained by emotionally detaching yourself from your loved one's problem. You will find a way to keep loving your partner, child, etc., without having to like their behavior around food. You will learn a way of being more interested, but less involved. The keystone is in letting this become more *their* problem and less *yours*. As long as you worry about their food behavior, *they don't have to*. The best way to help is to detach.

ENABLING PUNISHERS

Codependents travel quickly between extremes of enabling or punishing behaviors. One minute you might be overly protective, helpful, and conciliatory, and the next minute raging and criticizing and threatening abandonment. You try hard to be helpful because you want to "make a difference," "have an effect," "be worthwhile." When all efforts fail, you become punitive and enraged and demand immediate perfection. All your efforts at helping the E-D are a way to prove you are "okay," "nice people." If the E-D stays sick, you take this personally.

As attempts at controlling the eating continue to fail, you become disappointed and angry at the overeater's failed promises. You alternate between "understanding" the problem and quietly fuming with rage. You feel like they're doing it to *you*. The truth is that they are just doing it—and mostly to themselves, not you. You become a nagger and scolder, obsessed with watching another eat. You make comments about weight and diet to family and friends. This may be your way of excusing the eating and also showing you are actively working to do something about it. In truth, it's not your job!

In such relationships, difficulties develop when messages are unclear. Trying to effect a helpful, "enabling" image, you may actually be enraged, and, smiling icily through clenched teeth say, "You really don't want to eat that, do you dear?" Later, you get fed up with enabling and decide to crack down. You declare, "I'm sick and tired of putting up with paying your bills and watching you kill yourself. If this doesn't stop, I'm through!" Despite the speech, the check is written yet another time and threats to leave are idle. So no one believes what anyone else says, and the cycle continues.

MONITORS

Steve had spent years trying to help his wife Melinda with her problem. They had an agreement that he would monitor her weight. Each morning, Steve stood over Melinda as she weighed in on the bathroom scale. He carried a chart attached to a clipboard and diligently recorded each reading. Melinda gained 30 pounds during the first month of this plan. Steve's involvement promoted guilt and fear in Melinda. She coped with her rising anxiety by eating "at him."

Their case is not uncommon. Husbands often try to help with their wives' weight problems. They are actually the least likely person to be helpful; they are too personally involved and too invested in success. There is also often an unconscious fear about success which can work to sabotage their efforts.

In 1979, researchers at the University of Pennsylvania began to examine some of the investments husbands had in their wives' weight problems.

While the wives were enrolled in the University's weight control program, husbands were surveyed to determine their attitudes about the project. They were asked the following questions with interesting results:

1. Do you want to see your wife lose weight?
   Yes   50
   No   3
   Don't Care   2
2. Are you willing to assist your wife in losing weight?
   Yes   27
   No   17
   No Answer   11
3. Is your wife heavier now than when you were married?
   Yes   41
   No   8
   Same   6

(Notice how the numbers change in the first two questions. Nearly all the husbands wanted to see their wives lose weight, but when asked to offer help, their interest faltered. The answers to the fourth question are significant.)

4. *In your own words,* what changes would weight reduction by your wife mean to you?

Loss of eating as a shared activity	29
Loss of a bargaining position in arguments	27
Loss of wife in divorce	21
Worry about unfaithfulness	17

Notice how loss and fear permeate the responses. In their own words, these men were worried that they would: (1) lose a binge buddy; (2) lose the advantage of saying, "you fat slob, what do you know?" They anticipated not the joy of having an attractive spouse, but a fear that their wives' heightened self-image might destroy the relationship. She might have new options: divorce and infidelity. These men expressed more fear of loss than anticipated joy of success.

As a spouse, you are not the right helper to enlist in the weight loss game. Despite your best intentions, there may be too much at stake.

Other studies support the position that husbands usually exert a negative rather than positive influence on the wife's project. Couples enrolled in weight loss programs were observed through video and audio tapes to determine their behavior patterns around food. Even though wives were trying to take their attention off food, husbands constantly brought up food-relevant topics. They asked their wives seemingly insignificant questions about dinners and menus for no apparent reason. While eating together, the husbands were the ones most likely to keep offering extra helpings to their spouses. It was almost as if they were working very hard to show how truly lenient and "disinterested" they were. However, when wives did give in to eating, husbands were quick to blame and ridicule their wives' behavior. They rarely praised abstinent eating behaviors, but were quick to point out any slips in the food program.

Such studies lead us to postulate that loved ones want to see weight loss and success as long as they can control it. If they have involvement and can take credit, they will help, but if it is done by and for *self*, spouses may sabotage. This will be important throughout this book as you will see that sometimes family members feel they have more to lose than to gain, and thus will try to pull the E-D away from recovery programs.

The most helpful involvement from the spouse is to take a role of interested disinterest. You must show care and support but clearly give the message that what the E-D does, they are doing for themselves only! Keep your eyes on your own plate. More succinctly, it has to be a position of minding your own business.

VIVA LA COMPANY

Often, employers become the well-meaning monitors using established poundage standards, thus trying to control the eating.

Such techniques have never worked as a long-range solution. I have treated hundreds of flight attendants from major airlines which require weight checks for personnel. They set unrealistic standards of perfection, demanding that a forty-year-old flight attendant have the same weight as when she hired into the company at age twenty-two. (A few years ago, one major airline did move to institute a flexible schedule which allowed employees to gain three pounds each *decade!*) The idea that a scale determines competence is part of the problem.

The weighing-in procedure tends to promote sick leave abuses. The overweight flight attendant simply calls in sick during the weigh-in check week, then abuses amphetamines to control the eating and abuses laxatives to eliminate any effects. When she has reached her weight limit, she returns to record her poundage. As long as her weight is OK for that week, she's safe. Never mind the next month when she regains twenty pounds. Some have been so much over the weight limit that they are out months on sick leave with other "complaints," all the while abusing their bodies trying to comply with weight standards.

A compulsive eater facing the pressure of a weight check will perversely sabotage success by actually turning to food for solace. Annette had undergone four interviews before being chosen over a number of other highly qualified applicants for a civil service position. All that remained was a physical. Annette panicked. She knew she wouldn't qualify. She was relieved to find that, with her large frame, she only had two pounds to lose and a week to do it in order to get the job. Annette was hoping that, since she was not eating *meals*, the snacks wouldn't show and she'd get away with it. Instead she gained ten pounds! So much for weight checks.

DEATH WATCH

When efforts to monitor the weight of loved ones leave you exhausted, you can move into a *death watch* position. The daily bout with slow suicide leaves you feeling helpless. The feelings are similar to those of someone who cares for a chronically ill loved one. You see the daily sickness and don't dare hope for cure. This brings on depression. You may often isolate from the community. Seeing no clear-cut end to the suffering, you are in love with someone who is present in body but whose mind has left home long ago. You see a loved one seeking solace in food instead of you. This makes you angry, feeling abandoned, but you can't be angry with a sick person. Instead, you live in chronic anxiety and uncertainty, even at times wishing the E-D dead. That at least would be a clear end point with acceptable mourning rituals and an end to the suffering. With E-Ds it just seems like constant pain. Having wished the E-D dead, you feel guilty, so you overcompensate by being excessively helpful and loving. The anger erupts in power struggles and negotiation for control. The skirmishes often leave other innocents suffering from the fallout. Children often witness couples battling over control of food.

By the time I met Cassandra and Elliott, she weighed three hundred and he was addicted to a major tranquilizer to relieve his depression. Their marriage was stormy. From the very beginning, each fought for control. Her eating and his yard work were the overt issues. The power struggle progressed and she got fatter while the yard became a junk heap. Strangely enough, they came to see me because of their eight-year-old's bedwetting. The bedwetting was seen as the family problem.

As we talked, their depression emerged. Each felt they had failed the other. They were depressed, feeling they should be able to *do* something. When Elliott finally gave up on helping his wife lose weight, he became depressed. Pills helped him avoid. Each was watching the other die. The son knew no other way to show how helpless he felt than by wetting his bed. When Mom took responsibility for her own eating disorder, Dad stopped worrying about her and, instead, cleaned up the yard. He now sees hope in his wife's progress and is fulfilling his own responsibilities to his home and family. His depression is lifted. As a by-product of all this, Elliott, Jr. stopped wetting his bed.

HEALTHY NEUTRALITY

While overinvolvement with the sick person does not work, totally ignoring the problem doesn't work either. Healthy neutrality is when you care but don't take on the job. You are not attached to the outcome. You must learn to express your concern for them while letting them know your life will go on anyway. This kind of thinking may seem selfish and uncaring. Actually, it's a gift. You give up "fixing" someone and just let them know you love them whether they get "fixed" or not. You are starting to see that efforts at controlling and helping don't work. You need another way. That new way is giving up and letting go. This may sound easy, but is actually virtually impossible for a codependent alone. You must learn to say "no" and really mean it, and how to give the E-D's problem back to the one who really has it. In self-help groups you can discuss your own difficulties with other codependents. You will extend your family system to learn you are not alone. In later chapters, you'll see how to begin that learning.

"I ONLY HAVE EYES FOR YOU"

The codependent becomes a mirror image of the E-D, but the reflections become distorted. The codependent feels justified in taking over another person's life. E-Ds need codependents to tell them what to do. A codependent often assumes that he or she understands what the E-D is feeling better than the E-D. It is not uncommon to hear a codependent say, "I know what you're thinking." In response, the E-D will clam up or just cry. Quiet rebellion with food is not far behind. This reinforces the codependent's attitude that, "I must be right, they didn't even answer." So, both collude to promote the myth of incompetence on one hand, infallibility on the other. The E-D will silently fail while the codependent keeps trying and recommending new approaches. The codependent can maintain this fantasy indefinitely until the eating disorder eventually brings reality into focus. The codependent begins to wonder why this "well-controlled" person who "I fix" keeps gaining or losing weight. The E-D's body serves as a symbol of the futility of the codependent's efforts.

"WHY LOOK AT ME?"

A codependent's self-image is that of "giver" rather than "receiver." If you are a codependent, it is very difficult to accept the idea that you need help. Your questions will usually be something like the following.

What does this eating disorder have to do with me? If anything, I have only been trying to help this poor dear.
Didn't I offer to pay a dollar for each pound lost?
Didn't I offer to babysit while he or she went to those Weight Watcher meetings?
Didn't I buy a new wardrobe every time the body changed?
Didn't I gently remind about the diet every time he or she seemed to be slipping?
Didn't I help prepare all those special meals?
Didn't I support the gym membership that cost so much?

"How could someone suggest I'm the one who needs help?" Well, it *is* confusing. It is difficult to understand the point. Why would anyone want *you* to look at *yourself?* You wonder, "How can my self-examination in any way help the E-D?" That's a valid question and by the time you finish this book you will see that by becoming interested in your own life and taking care of yourself, the E-D will in turn assume more responsibility for his or her own life. You will both develop healthier mutual dependence and independence.

Whether you are in the position of spouse, friend, mother, daughter, sister, brother, father, employer, concerned professional, or just interested observer, your experience has a certain recognizable pattern. You have watched someone you care about become more and more obsessed with food, and more removed from you. You have watched a slow suicide. You've been affected. You are another victim of the disease. Your interest in the problem moves to an obsession in and of itself. The following graph shows the gradual progression of a codependent personality. Let's look at how you got here.

PROGRESSION OF CODEPENDENT PERSONALITY

Use this as a checklist to monitor your own progression.

EARLY STAGES

_____ Often born of dysfunctional family and learned to "care" for others as measure of self-worth.

_____ Failed to cure parents so will "cure" E-D.

_____ Finds E-D who is "needy" so controls.

_____ Begins doubting own perceptions and wants to control eating to show decisiveness.

_____ Social life affected. Isolates self from community to "help" E-D.

OBSESSION

_____ Makes pleas and threats related to the eating behavior.

_____ Judges self and feels the cause of eating/starving.

_____ Hides food.

_____ Attempts controlling eating, hiding food, idle threats, nagging, scolding.

_____ Shows anger and disappointment regarding E-D's promises.

SECRET LIFE

_____ Becomes obsessed with watching and covering up.

_____ Takes over responsibilities of E-D.

_____ Takes pivotal role in communications, excluding contact between E-D and others.

_____ Expresses anger inappropriately.

OUT OF CONTROL

_____ Makes violent attempts to control eating. Fights with E-D.

_____ Lets self go physically and mentally.

_____ Has extramarital affairs such as infidelity, workaholism, obsession with outside interests.

_____ Becomes rigid, possessive. Appears angry most of time and careful and secretive about home life.

_____ Has related illness and drug abuse: ulcers, rashes, migraines, depression, obesity, tranquilizers.

_____ Constantly loses temper.

_____ Becomes sick and tired of being sick and tired.

DEVELOPING CODEPENDENCY

Just as no one asks to have an eating disorder, you didn't ask to be a codependent either. No one questions that you came by it honestly and that you did the best you could with what you knew. You tried your best. Your intentions have been well-meant and your efforts genuine. Let's take a look at how your involvement developed.

Heredity. People with an eating disorder learned to use food to relieve stress long before they had any choice about it. Similarly, you learned to become a "caretaker" long before having any conscious choice. As a codependent you may have been born to a somewhat dysfunctional family who abused alcohol or other substances. You learned early to feel responsible for the pain of your parents. This mistaken sense of responsibility is the clearest indicator of codependency. Young children feel omnipotent, and consequently, responsible for the well-being of their parents. They feel they have created everything that happens around them. Children see themselves as the center of the universe. (Some carry this to adulthood.) In an addicted family, parents are suffering, and children, of course, take responsibility for the suffering. You may have even heard parents complain, "My life would have been much better without you kids." Or, a mother, after she is beaten by her alcoholic husband cries, "I would leave the SOB if it weren't for you children." You can see how a child would automatically take on guilt. If you come from such a family, your mission was programmed long before you ever thought about it.

Caretaker Role. In such families, you rarely learned to *expect* nurturing for yourself. You never learned how to *receive.* You learned to take care of others. As you see it, the degree to which you demonstrate caring and helpfulness is the measure of your own self-worth. You have not "cured" your parents' lives, so you're a failure. Their problems continued and progressed despite your best efforts. With your mission still unaccomplished, you need to find suffering persons and help them; this will be your redemption. Many people who become doctors, psychologists, social workers and nurses do so to try and make up for childhood failures. Marrying an E-D is another attempt.

Marry to Fix. Failing to cure your parents, you found a needy mate. The agenda then is to cure your spouse. You are still trying to win that badge by fixing *someone* you love. Taking on this mission keeps you feeling somewhat in control. In truth, however, you can't control them at all. Eating disorders have nothing to do with you, just like in the situation with your parents. It doesn't matter what you try or don't try. To marry a "needy" mate keeps you from ever having to face your own needs. You say you want to be the "receiver" but really don't know how. You may complain, "Why isn't it ever my turn to be the 'falling apart' person?" This lament is easily voiced where you know you won't be heard. Your relationship with an E-D keeps you deprived but safe.

Control is the Key. As the eating disorder progresses, you have usually escalated attempts at control. Initially this is effected with gentle pleadings to cut down. When this fails, the next step is subtle threats or promised rewards. "I'll pay you five dollars for every pound you lose." "Get into that new bathing suit and we'll go on a cruise." When such efforts produce no new results, you begin judging yourself as inadequate. Since you took on someone to fix, your ego and identity are very much tied to that person's success. If he or she fails, you fail. Fearful of the impending failure, you may escalate your threats, even threatening to leave. The E-D may turn the tables on you and also threaten to leave. At that point, you may often beg him or her to stay. You are recreating the same struggle you took on as a child: making a stand and then backing off. First helpful, then punitive, then guilty. Efforts escalate to hiding food, locking cabinets, nagging, and scolding. No matter what efforts you undertake, the eating disorder moves ahead of you.

Pivotally Pissed Off. The E-D has made and broken innumerable promises. Despite whatever appropriate, caring, "helpful benefactor" feelings you'd like to effect, the truth is that you are angry. Often you have taken over many of the E-D's responsibilities. Initially you took on these extra burdens as a labor of love. It felt good to be giving. However, you expected this would be temporary and you later began to resent the permanence of your benefactor role. You may be the "family message center," becoming overburdened and involved in everyone's business. Whatever problems exist in the family, you wish the E-D would handle his or her share.

You have seen the E-D through inappropriate and widely varying mood swings based on whether they are on a binge or in withdrawal. You wanted to protect others from some of this so you became the communication hub for everyone; interpreting and rephrasing all conversations so no one would be hurt. "Mommy's having a bad day. She didn't mean it." Unfortunately, this role hurts you. If you are busy analyzing and heading off others' emotions, you will never have a chance to acknowledge and feel your own. Most of the time, you won't even notice the toll this takes on you.

Sometimes your rage comes out in the form of ulcers, colitis, migraines, or other physical complaints. However, as time moves on, you will have to express pent-up resentment at this role. After brewing underground for so long, your anger may surface inappropriately in a way which is embarrassing or humiliating. Codependents often look angry all the time, but no one knows why. After all, the E-D has been walking around partially sedated while you have faced all the family problems coldly and soberly conscious. You didn't have the comfort of food abuse! You may effect the "silent treatment" for a while, only to eventually falter into loud and hostile outbursts when least expected. Embarrassed and guilty from such outbursts, you may become excessively apologetic and walk on eggshells to smooth over your recent behavior. In this way, the codependent and the E-D mirror each other. Both feel guilty, out of control, frustrated and angry. Both compensate by becoming overly conciliatory and apologetic. Such behavior merely perpetuates the problem.

Who Cares? "If ya can't beat 'em, join 'em! Caring, not caring, raging, silencing, hinting, cajoling, nagging, scolding . . . NOTHING WORKS." You hang on precariously as the pendulum swings between rigid silence and maniacal ravings. You live with insecurity and without hope for the future. You don't know what kind of behavior to expect from your E-D or yourself, and all the while you have an image of yourself as being able to keep things in control. The only solution is to give up trying. Often you have let your own grooming and personal care slack off. "If they don't care, why should I?" You may decide to join your E-D and develop your own form of substance abuse. In an informal survey, I discovered at least 40 percent of the wives of alcoholics were obese. Codependents also become addicted to sedatives and tranquilizers (all doctor-prescribed) as alternatives to anxiety.

RUN AWAY FROM HOME

The runaway problem in such homes is not merely packing up and moving on. The codependent leaves by withdrawing emotional investment and finding outside activities to gain satisfaction. This is actually a healthy survival adjustment. Although it weakens the family structure, leaving is the only way to endure a situation in which you have no effect. Tests done with monkeys have dramatized this point. Monkeys were alternately shocked and rewarded with no possibility of figuring out which response would come when. No matter what they tried, there was no escape. Eventually, the monkeys stopped trying at all. Later, when new options were offered, they sat in a helpless, hopeless huddle, refusing to try. This is termed "learned helplessness" and beautifully characterizes the codependent personality. You withdraw to survive.

If you don't withdraw and close down completely, you may decide to gain personal satisfaction outside the home. Since your own self worth is tied to helping someone, you will have to become a helper away from home. At home you still feel like a total failure. You may become a "workaholic." As you work twelve to fourteen hour days, you can finally say, "I've done enough." You may decide to become president of the Chamber of Commerce or PTA, or a scout leader, thus gaining recognition and approval from others.

The more the home situation fails, the more you throw yourself into these outside projects. Often the E-D may suspect infidelity, but that is rarely the case. Actually, you still won't even feel good enough about yourself to allow for an affair.

Sick and Tired of Being Sick and Tired. You reached being fed up long ago. When you are sick and tired of being sick and tired, you are ready to take positive action to effect some change. Here you reach the same crisis point as the E-D where you say, "My God, this is really my life, not a drill! Not a dress rehearsal! I have to listen and learn a new way." Some think of a quick, runaway solution such as a divorce. This is rarely effective. Guilt lingers, and the mutual nature of the disease is never addressed. More than likely you would remarry into the same situation. You must learn about your own role in such a predicament. It is imperative that you address whatever personal needs you have in this type of relationship. If you don't, you will continue the cycle yet another time. You may as well work through it here.

Chapter Four

Why Are We Together?

One E-D keeps fifteen to twenty codependents busy. You are each an extension of the other. You each take on opposite sides of the same personality structure. While the E-D falls apart, a codependent tries to put things back together. Both together constitute one fully functioning adult human being. Trading off the roles presents problems. Roles will alternate. Food determines who fits where in the equation. When food makes an E-D super-achieving and functional, codependents benefit from the energy. Other times, food creates self-loathing, depression and angry, irrational outbursts. Then the codependent becomes comforter, rescuer. As the obsessive use of food to cope with life increases, it becomes more and more difficult to predict the effects of the eating. Giving up the food often creates a total personality change. Let's just say that at this point food no longer works as a coping mechanism. Continual return to it gets nowhere, and you can't predict what effects are in store. You do know however, that you are "sick and tired of being sick and tired." You are ready to find a new way out. This is the beginning of recovery.

"AS IF" PERSONALITY

To give up food you must renegotiate your place in the world. It is no accident that you have taken on an illness which allows your physical body to undulate intermittently. Your inner self is trying to establish its own place, and it is confused about how large or small it wants to be and how much space it needs to take up. Your "honest" self is looking for its true home. When you take on unrealistic roles for yourself, your body signals your personal deceit. "The body doesn't lie. The head does."

You fashioned yourself in such a way that you thought you could achieve love and closeness and instead lost *yourself* in the process. Fat is the price paid for love. Most often, this trade-off for love occurred first in the mother-child relationship. You took the patterns you learned there with you into adulthood. Needing love as well as needing independence, you struggle with a fear of being trapped as well as a longing to be swallowed up. You can avoid that struggle as long as you keep swallowing up every piece of food in sight. When the eating obsession stops, you will start to see how much of yourself you have traded off in order to play the roles that would win you love.

PRISONERS OF CHILDHOOD

Early research with obese families was conducted by psychiatrist Hilde Bruch in the 1940s. She found that mothers of obese children were often insecure and had ambivalence regarding the child. They weren't sure if they really wanted the child or not. Often the child was born late in life and wasn't really planned for or expected. Even today it is still taboo for mothers to express anything less than exultation at having a child. There is great fear the child will be damaged emotionally, as if the child doesn't already know anyway.

Upset at their own mixed emotions, these mothers compensate by excessive feeding and extreme overprotectiveness. They want to insure that the child feels loved. The food would offer the security and satisfaction they feared they could not give. To prove how much love was there, they made the children clinging and dependent. They inhibited the children from risk-taking and muscular activity. The mothers were often "sick" themselves. Whenever the children presented needs the parent hadn't planned for, the mother had her own complaints, usually competing to show "who is sicker."

The fathers in these homes were either absent or weak and unaggressive. They were treated by their wives with a great deal of contempt and reproach. The wives, being "sickly types," did a lot of blaming of Dad, and berated him constantly. The message to the child was, "No matter what, don't be like your father." This dynamic operates in overeating women. Many have great struggles with men's strength and their own. They want a strong man, but also fear him. Even more, they become fearful when showing their own strengths. They don't want to intimidate anyone.

Growing up, these children were not very close with their fathers. They felt like possessions of the father. He was more interested in work or business activities. Despite business acclaim, his efforts never achieved him acclaim within the family system. Even if the dad had been successful in a business area, it was never enough. Mom continued to complain that "her" needs were not met.

In further research, a number of fathers' occupations were predicted to produce fat daughters. The top three occupations were dress manufacturer, movie producer, and specialist in metabolic diseases. It was almost as if the daughters decided not to compete. If what Daddy wanted was thin model types, beautiful movie stars, or great successes from his medical practice, the daughters absolutely insisted on being the opposite.

BREAKING THE TIE THAT BINDS

Despite your early programming, you'll have to struggle to grow up and leave home. When you truly reach an adult commitment to live your own life, the food obsession will take on a whole different character. This is true whether you have moved three thousand miles away from home or live around the block. It is true if you are a teenage anorexic struggling to grow up in high school or a forty-year-old mother of four who presents herself as "earth mother" to everyone but herself. Recovering from the eating disorder is a definite statement that you will begin to live your own life for yourself. This is it.

Even if you are married and geographically separated from your mother, the emotional struggle to separate is the crucial one for your recovery. If your separation plans don't work out well, attachment to food often results. Often the marriage contract is a new commitment to the same old struggle you have with leaving Mom's home. You may have married your mother. You marry the same struggle you had with Mom. For example, if at home you usually felt guilty, as if you had never done enough, you may well marry someone who helps you feel guilty, as though you don't measure up. If, at Mom's home, you felt superior and special and spoiled, you will marry someone who keeps that fantasy going. If you felt inadequate and competitive in childhood, you will likely marry into the same situation. In any event, you will need to find new ways to relate in order to recover.

MUTUAL DEPENDENCY

Though E-Ds and codependents complain about each other, you are more alike than you are different. You are, in a very real sense, *mirror images* of each other. One takes on one extreme, and the other its opposite. There is nothing inherently wrong with this, in fact many people thrive on this interdependency. With eating disorders however, the addition of food into the equation upsets the balance. The personality dynamics are common to many people, whether or not they exhibit any form of addiction. Most people can function quite well without examining their relationships. E-Ds and their codependents, however, have to look at relationship patterns. The only other alternative is to keep food obsessions in the picture.

You have been using food to avoid risk. You have failed to explore and "own" all parts of your personality. You stayed with what was safe. In choosing partners, you gravitated to people who could fulfill the parts of you that you feared. If you feared being aggressive, you chose someone to act that out for you. If you feared being too braggardly, you chose someone to be shy for you. Whatever you are avoiding will have to be faced in recovery.

From time to time you may undergo role reversals as you each try on new parts of yourself. As you both recover, you will each become more functional as separate individuals. As relationships with people become healthier, the relationship with food will, too. Food was used to avoid the risk of growing into full adulthood. Now let's see what emerged and what was left behind in your adult personality.

EXTREMISM

As I said earlier, E-Ds and their codependents gravitate toward opposite personality traits, becoming rigidly fixed in one mode or the other. These people are both attracted to, and repulsed by, their opposites. They work well together to keep conflict and control in the foreground. When they are busy trying to change the other, they have no time left to experiment with a more moderate position for themselves. By focusing on the other person they ignore themselves. Healthy recovery involves developing your personalities so as to have options about which behaviors to take on when. With new behavior options, you will move closer to your center. It is not always worthwhile to be the outgoing life of the party, nor is it always essential to be neat and well-groomed. You will practice becoming your opposite. This kind of change is difficult, especially when certain learned behaviors seem to work well and help you survive. You must melt a little. This makes you more alive, and you won't need food for sedation. As natural cells constantly fuse and separate, so human relationships need the same fluidity. By staying fixated and obsessed, you became unable to weather movement and change. Recovery is change! You grow or you go.

REACTORS

Each of you E-Ds reacts to external cues rather than internal motivation. Research has shown the E-Ds tend to be externally-oriented individuals. You are highly responsive to outer stimuli, but very vague on messages from your own bodies. In studies, obese and "normal" subjects were asked to go into a room and then report what they saw. Normal people reported seeing, "a chair, a desk, and a lamp." Obese subjects reported elaborate details of "a blue tweed chair, a Victorian desk, a picture on the wall with an autumnal scene, blue specked wallpaper, etc." E-Ds are highly sensitized to the environment and react to what comes towards them. In doing math problems, their performance diminished when music was played. Normal people continued at the same level despite external stimuli. E-Ds are thrown off base by externals more easily than normal subjects. Similarly, E-Ds tend to respond to external expectations. Placed in a room with no windows, but with a clock, E-Ds reported hunger and expected lunch when the clock showed noon, even though the time was actually 9:30 A.M. Normal people reported with dismay that they "didn't feel like eating even though it was 'lunch time.'" They responded to *internal* stimuli.

Codependents, though not as responsive to food cues, are very sensitized to the feelings of others. If you have a splinter, the codependent's finger might hurt. This trait is an asset in "helping profession" careers, but can be anathema in a personal relationship. Constantly reacting to the needs of another allows little chance to develop a sensitivity to one's own needs. Remember how codependents tend to come from families with addictive parents? They develop an ability to watch closely and gauge another's feelings. They have learned to walk on eggshells, to be overly helpful and sympathetic as a way of warding off criticism. They learned little in the way of making positive, assertive stands for themselves. They have difficulty receiving and are more comfortable giving. Both E-Ds and codependents are highly responsive to others and too little in touch with themselves. Therefore, they each need to have the other around as a base from which to react.

PASSIVE/AGGRESSIVE STRUGGLES

If one is the tough guy, the bully, the other will be fragile and dependent. "You wear the white hat, I'll take the black one." Two fairly typical patients in hospital treatment are Passive Pauline and Aggressive Angela. The passive one wants to be wheeled in on a gurney with intravenous tubes in each arm. She wants to lie back and say "Wake me when it's over." She wants no active part in her recovery. "Just fix me," she says. She may warn the treatment staff that her case is so difficult that there is actually no cure possible! This is "terminal uniqueness." Passive Pauline presents passivity and dependency as a challenge. "Prove to me, Doc, that you will make the difference."

Passive individuals teach a well-meaning codependent to try and "make the difference." While the more aggressive helper assumes the rescuer role, Pauline stays rigidly locked into passivity. Both are convinced that one is a "failure" and the other a "fixer." Without a codependent, the passive person can't fall totally to pieces. It takes two.

Aggressive Angela is just the opposite. She enters treatment aggressive and boisterous. She explains to everyone that she knows what works and what doesn't. She tells us how to fix her. She begins with a highly critical and judgmental evaluation of the treatment team, then moves quickly to become a co-therapist and colleague of the therapy group leader. She has great difficulty receiving and being in a nurtured position. She has to grieve at giving up control. Much as she longs to be cared for, it is safer to be giving. (Often such patients are nurses. They have found a profession which helps them maintain their giver role, but often keeps them fat.)

This aggressive person usually attaches to someone who is needy. She will avoid people who give because they are a much greater risk. When she gives up the food obsession she becomes needy and must learn how to receive. She will also start expecting more from the people she once helped.

EGO STRUGGLES

Often called "egomaniacs with inferiority complexes," E-Ds and codependents have little sense of real personal worth. It is easier and safer to be reflecting others. It is a constant comparison game. Who am I? Compared to what? You seek out "better than" or "less than" relationships, but can rarely tolerate one based on equality. Food gets abused in the process of maintaining the power balance. If, as an "inferior" person, you start feeling too good, you use the food to get back in position again. If you were in the superior position, you may need to fall apart a little. You will expect your opposite to rise to the occasion. Recovery involves assuming an image of yourself that has nothing to do with someone else's success or failure. But you must gain a realistic picture of yourself. This leads to being free to love without a power struggle. In healthy relating you will exalt in being ordinary.

ANGER BLOCKERS

I have not met an E-D yet who was not raging within. E-Ds use food to push down anger. You judge anger as highly inappropriate. Perhaps you saw inappropriate expressions of anger in childhood and are afraid to repeat the pattern. Rather than confronting an angry situation directly, you smile ingratiatingly and seethe within. Codependents can exhibit the same avoidance of anger and quietly withdraw rather than air legitimate grievances. Recovery involves acknowledging your anger and then telling someone else. You don't necessarily have to confront the object of your anger directly. You might vent enough by confiding in others. If you are an anger blocker, you choose angry friends who talk *for* you. E-Ds may express a codependent's anger so that he or she can maintain a "nice guy" image. Food supplies energy to be angry. Giving up food may make you less willing to fight the old battles.

HOPELESSNESS CYCLE

Why be angry? E-Ds and codependents have years of failed attempts at controlling the food obsession. You have lowered your expectations and have lost your motivation to take on anything new. This hopelessness must be expressed and acknowledged before recovery can begin. You played out an elaborate game, one sad, the other happy-go-lucky. This works as long as each stays in character, but what happens when the long-suffering fat housewife says she will "go for it, no matter what," and is genuinely motivated and energized to develop a new life? What happens when she takes over the happy role? Where does that leave the codependent? Getting happy will upset the system. Often people don't want to hope again because they are afraid of change.

MAGICAL THINKING

One sure fire way to remain hopeless is to believe in magic. Magical thinking helps you remain a victim of the "weight loss, diet fad" mentality. You buy all the books and pills that promise an instant cure. In a way, you desperately want to believe they work, and they sometimes do—for brief periods. Since your body changed form so rapidly, it is easy to think your life could change just as easily. Even though thinner, you found problems you couldn't solve, and you returned to the abuse of food, and made that your problem again. That at least has a magic solution!

PERFECTIONISM

Well, since we can't control food, let's at least make sure everything else is perfect. It seems easier to be perfect in business, house cleaning, childrearing, etc., than dealing with the food obsession. Both E-Ds and codependents run coworkers, friends, and family ragged to maintain standards of perfection. They hope to mask their feelings of failure with regard to food. If not playing "perfect success," you may play "perfect failure." It takes just as much effort to fail as it does to "go for it."

LOW FRUSTRATION TOLERANCE

Perfection means "do it my way faster." You must maintain highly ritualized standards of how things should operate, especially when it comes to how others should perform. To keep control of the situation, and especially the outcome, you devise elaborate scripts detailing where, how, and when people should speak, move, or breathe. When others don't perform to expectations, it is extremely irritating.

Many tell me, "You're wrong here! If there is one thing I can endure, it is frustration." They brag about the business and professional situations in which they keep a cool, corporate exterior. They did that with food! Without the abuse of food, irritability rapidly rises. Excess food has enabled you to maintain serenity while others panicked. Without food, you may be the Captain of Chaos. If you can keep your head while those around you are losing theirs, perhaps you don't adequately understand the situation.

MORALISTIC ATTITUDES

Another aspect of perfectionism is to maintain an impossibly high standard of morality for yourself and others. E-Ds and codependents often enter into fierce philosophical discussions about morality. You can maintain excessive standards as long as you keep shoveling the food in. Perhaps the codependent is living out the opposite side of this equation, balancing immorality to the tune of the E-D's morality. Maybe the E-D is a secret seductress and afraid to get thin to find out. In recovery, this also is renegotiated. Obese women, fearful that losing weight will cause them to go raping and pillaging through the streets, stay fat and celibate and leave the runaround role for others. They are satisfied to sit in judgment.

ALL-OR-NOTHING MENTALITY

Nothing gradual or moderate gets attention in E-D relationships. The complaint with recovery is, "Serenity is boring." To reach "higher highs" and correspondingly "lower lows," the E-D and code-pendent keep balanced. Either you are rigidly stuck on an abusive, restrictive food plan, or you eat the refrigerator and then some. With the perfectionistic expectation operating anyway, you will trans-pose it to food and use any deviation as an excuse to binge. The dieting mentality feeds right into this problem. Ritualized prescriptions of what to eat create dogged adherence followed by rejection of the whole plan and return to bingeing. I am constantly amused to read that "one cup of popped popcorn contains 55 calories." Does anyone eat only one cup of popcorn? How about the calorie count for a *tub* of buttered popcorn? E-Ds don't eat one cup. Who does? Why bother?

WORKAHOLICS

Perhaps if you work hard enough and succeed, your professional accomplishments will camouflage your eating disorder. This is surely the wish of many young career women; rapid achievers in a competi-tive world who binge and vomit nightly. Professional success in one area makes up for the lack of control in another. Often, the worka-holic will be a codependent, who, failing to cure their spouse or child, tries to prove him- or herself in other areas to feel accomplished. In recovery, many workaholics become just average, so-so workers. No longer needing to prove themselves or cover up food obsessions, they begin to put in an honest day for an honest dollar, no more and no less. This can present problems at work, where your employer enjoyed the fruits of your obsession. That person may try to recreate the old system!

PEOPLE PLEASERS

Just so no one will say anything about your weight problem, you might decide to be the nice guy at all costs. If others enjoy your company, they will excuse your appearance, or so goes the rationale. E-Ds and codependents learn to anticipate the needs of others and fit in. You become chameleons, adapting to the needs of others. In your own relating, one may take on being the "sweet-heart" while the other plays "sullen grouch." The people pleaser keeps excusing and explaining the behavior of the grouch. Unfortunately, your own feelings in the situation get pushed down with food.

FEAR OF SUCCESS

Despite being excessive workaholics and superachievers, E-Ds and codependents fear success. A large reason for this is the fear that, if successful, you will have to maintain it. Remember your standards of perfection! If your true capabilities are known, you fear you will be expected to perform at maximum efficiency at all times. Since you can't possibly achieve your own standard, it's easier not to succeed. This fear of success holds true with weight loss. Many get down to within ten pounds of goal weight and start back up again. In recovery you learn to tolerate "progress, not perfection" and accept the fact that, even though successful, you will have bad days. "Big girls *do* cry."

FEAR OF INTIMACY

You both fear intimacy for the same reason you fear success. You can't endure the expectation that you might have to maintain it. You think true intimacy involves eyeball to eyeball seriousness and deep catharsis or sharing. Who would want to stay locked in that? Even the most dramatic intimate scenes in a movie last but a few seconds. Who could tolerate more? Just as cells in nature come together and divide, so your closeness needs the same ebb and flow. You might feel cuddly and close one day and the next each go to separate rooms to read the paper. What's wrong with that? In *The Prophet*, Kahlil Gibran advises, "allow for spaces in your together- ness."

ISOLATIONISTS

With so many conflicts about intimacy, distance, achieving, fail- ing, working, quitting, anger, and pleasing, it is no wonder E-Ds and codependents would rather be alone. At least alone you have no one's expectations but your own. Unfortunately, as your eating disorder progresses, it becomes less and less tolerable to be alone. There is too much guilt and self-loathing and worry. The only relief from overactive self-loathing is associated with food. Eventually, however, food also stops working. E-Ds and codependents often isolate themselves among others like them, but it only makes the situation worse to join together in denial and depression.

The way out is through people, but not just anybody. It is easy to win friends and influence people by being helpers and people pleasers. You can find people who will "like" you very much. That's not what you need. If that had helped, you wouldn't be in the food now. You've actually been winning these new friends through chameleon-like adaptation rather than representing who you really are. To "relate to recover," you need a way to talk and be heard. In Marilyn French's book, *The Women's Room,* she explains, "Loneliness is not a longing for company. It's a longing for *kind.*" E-Ds and codependents find their kind in meetings of Overeaters Anonymous and O-Anon. This is where you can talk and be heard. With your kind, you can share the pain and suffering of an eating disorder, find comfort, and then move on. You will be able to show the real person inside instead of the "act as if" with food.

TRADING ROLES FOR REALITIES

There's more to lose than fat. There's also much more to gain than just a fleeting thinness. When your relationships change you won't want to go back to the old system. You won't even be able to. Those old stereotyped roles will seem boring to you. Let's take a look at the old roles and the new approaches which lead out of addiction.

The Victim.　This is the starring role for our fat family's drama. Without the continued suffering of the E-D, everyone else is quickly displaced. That is partly why the E-D has to keep suffering. By suffering, you are insuring that those around you remain secure and protected. The victim, though hurting, is a subtle blamer. "You made me this way. You have to fix me." There is a great deal of strength in failing. Just by the law of averages, you are bound to succeed 50 percent of the time. If you continue to fail regularly, you must be working at it. Thus, there is great unleashed power and energy held by the victim. The victim's blaming is never too direct, as that would reveal too much strength. Instead, the victim shows continual self-loathing and guilt as a way to deny personal possibilities for happiness. This also keeps everyone else in the family working to fix her. Thank God she stays sick! In this way, she is the family scapegoat. All can complain, "We'd be happy if only _____ would get it together." If the E-D does not continue this role, someone else in the family will take it on. This person is actually a family hero, and serves as the excuse to not fly.

As long as the E-D continues to suffer, other family members (codependents) won't have to test their own capacities for happiness. To recover, you codependents will have to find your *own* way, whether you "cured" the E-D or not. You will have to take personal responsibility for yourselves.

The former victim used to complain, "I'm a hopeless failure and just won't ever make it."

The recovering victim now declares, "Today I'm doing the best I can. At least I'm getting started and that's all I can manage today."

The Enabler. If the victim holds star billing in this drama, the enabler is certainly the most important supporting character. Enablers wear the white hats while E-Ds don the black ones (in the mind of the enabler, of course). As an enabler, you provide stability in an unstable system. You are great organizers, workers, and successes in business. You promptly do chores or whatever else is asked. As children, you do well in school, exhibiting strong leadership qualities, and are usually highly goal oriented, known as being realistic and rational minds. Outwardly, you espouse feelings of high self-esteem, but you rarely develop intimate personal relationships. In that area, you don't quite feel worthwhile. If asked to give up rigid control or open boundaries to others you will become fearful. It's safer to control by helping. With only slight encouragement from the E-D, you move in to take on the whole job of recovery. You will need to move out of the way so the E-D can fall apart if they have to. Let them sink or swim on their own. They are not your responsibility.

The former enabler used to say, "I refused the party invitation because I knew you couldn't handle the food."

The recovering enabler now declares, "Your friend Jane phoned about the restaurant party. I figured you'd know how you want to handle it. She's waiting for your call back."

Persecutor. The persecutor role is usually played by a parent or spouse. This role serves the dual function of helping the victim remain sick, and at the same time blaming them for being sick. It is a double message. You rescue and cajole the E-D for a certain amount of time. Then patience runs out and you begin to criticize and demand perfection. Like the buzzards perched atop a dried cactus branch, you finally scream, "The hell with patience. I want to kill something!" The one to kill is the E-D, and though not actually killing, your rage lies just below the surface. These feelings are usually masked with a thin veil of "helpful" manipulations. Though critical, the enabler is also the constant "pusher," encouraging a binge "just this once." There is great pain suffered in this dual personality. You have to find a way to express anger directly. You must first reject the eating disorder. The message to the E-D will be, "I love *you,* but hate your *disease.* I won't support this self-destructive behavior any longer. You've got your troubles, I've got mine. I give up on fixing you."

Once you voice this position, be quiet. You don't need to keep haranguing and you don't need to move in to help. Speak your piece and back off.

You will have to find a way to forgive yourself for your old punitive stands. You really don't like yourself that way, but you have responded to the frustrations of your own powerlessness. The best way to forgive yourself is to begin immediately to change your behavior. No elaborate speeches are needed. No declarations of future perfection are called for.

The former persecutor used to say, "You are a weak-willed glutton and you disgust me."

The recovering persecutor now says, "It hurts me to watch your suffering. You'll have to do that alone."

Persecutors and enablers want some appreciation for all the effort they've expended. You had hoped you could shame the E-D into shaping up. Instead, the illness got worse.

One of the saddest families I've treated came to my attention as the overeater/alcoholic mother was admitted to our hospital's emergency room with lacerations of the face and neck. Upon later investigation, we found the mother had promised her twelve-year-old daughter, Emily, that she was beginning a diet and going on the wagon. That afternoon, upon returning from school, Emily found her mother passed out in the kitchen lying among cracker and chip boxes along with an empty bottle of bourbon. In her rage and frustration, she beat her mother; eventually being pulled off by an older brother. Imagine the pain this daughter feels from both loving and hating her E-D mother! In this case, the daughter needs help in accepting her rage and forgiving herself as a fellow victim of the illness.

Emily had previously taken over management of the household because Mom was too nervous and "suffering" to handle her own responsibilities. Daughter, Emily, was the enabler as well as the persecutor. Emily likes managing but hates it, too. She will have to learn to be a child again rather than Mommy's mommy. She'll also have to forgive Mommy for not being well enough before. She has to give up wanting to be paid back. She'll have to seek her own payback.

The Clown. "Let me make a joke of myself before you do." "At all costs, let's keep things light." "Why make a big deal of everything?" "Why so serious?" The clown can be either an E-D or a codependent. Clowns see the family's suffering and develop themselves as a form of diversion. They are quick, witty, and fun to be around. They laugh and play and pretend life is light. They espouse "devil may care, c'est la vie" attitudes, but are actually closely tuned to the suffering. They are reactors rather than actors for themselves. Joking or distracting, they pretend they are irrelevant; just hanging around for comic relief.

As a clown, you have seen the chaotic addicted family system and decided not to play. You create distractions to help the family avoid intimacy. Acting uninvolved, you approach a heated family battle and ask innocently, "Are we going to the beach next Saturday?" You hope such distractions help others avoid pain. You see intimacy as death. Denying intimacy, you don't know how to take yourself seriously. Often developing your own alternate addiction is the only way to relax, or be taken seriously. You have spent so much time distracting that you have become distracted from yourself.

The former clown used to spoof, "I'm such a tub o'lard; I know I'll break the chair."

The recovering clown now says, "I feel badly about my situation. I need to talk and be heard."

The Hero. Often a sibling, fellow worker, or spouse, the hero decides to excel and achieve to prove that all is well. You try to cover up suffering. You appear sensitive and insightful and aware of others as well as feeling extremely responsible. You push to achieve and accomplish in order to make things better for everyone. In recovery, you may have to learn how to fall apart. When you move aside, you create room for the "failing" E-D to show his or her stuff and measure up. When the hero dominates the success spot, the E-D stays sick so as not to displace anyone.

The former hero used to brag, "Don't worry Scarlett. I'll be here ever-ready to solve your problems."

The recovering hero now says, "It's really up to you. I've got better things to do. Frankly Scarlett. . . ."

The Recluse. At all costs, make no waves! The quiet and shy recluse senses the anxiety and fear of the family and decides to withdraw in order to avoid contributing to the family's suffering. You feel the family suffers enough and want to shrivel up to have no effect. If you withdraw, you feel successful. Often the recluse is a child who spends much time alone, demanding little attention, inviting comments like, "At least this is the one child I don't have to worry about." You learned that family involvement revolves around sickness. Not knowing how to play sick, you'd rather not play at all. In recovery, you will have to discover new personal excitement and learn to have fun. You have to release the energy you've been holding back and risk having an impact on others. You can't avoid it. You *do* exist and you *do* have an effect.

The withdrawn recluse used to project, saying, "Don't consider me. I'll make my own way."

The recovering recluse takes action by saying, "Count me in. I'm to be considered also."

The Survivors. All members of this system have learned to adjust and survive. Some have even developed suffering into a badge of courage or martyrdom. You all know how to adjust. You've learned to be compliant and amenable to others. Great at following directions, you may also seek employment that offers constant uncertainty (commission sales or publishing deadlines). You know how to anticipate the needs of others, and adapt with chameleon-like rapidity. Underneath all the surviving is deep depression and loneliness because you never learned to represent your true selves. You try at all costs to avoid expressing feelings. Expressing feelings rarely got anything but criticism. When sad, no comfort was available. When angry, you were punished. When expressing yourself, you were usually ignored. You learned to adjust and manipulate others, but ultimately lost yourself.

SERENITY IS BORING

Without help, such family members drift further apart into their separate isolation and loneliness. The system survives as long as the addiction is operating. Everyone has silently, and often unconsciously, made compromises to the disease process. Often, the family has become isolated from the community. Party invitations have been refused, public functions are avoided, and children's school activities aren't supported. People have developed the attitude that it doesn't matter. Husbands tell themselves, "I really didn't want to go to the party anyway." Children sigh, "It's really not important if Mom comes along." Sexually frustrated husbands protest that perhaps they are too demanding and need to give their spouses rest. After her binge, she lies passed out on the couch. Family members begin to doubt their own perceptions: "Did Mom really promise to take me to the park, or did I make it up?" "I thought for sure she said she wanted to go to the store." "Why is she just sitting there eating?"

This family has adjusted to a chaotic situation. They live in constant uncertainty. They do not know how to live calmly. Violent contact was seen as an expression of caring and involvement. Calmness in recovery is taken as withdrawal and lack of love. Family members sometimes try to recreate the old conflicts so that they will feel involved and close again. They sometimes complain that the situation has become boring at home. What do they share in common now? The opposite situation can also exist. If, while eating, the overeater tended to withdraw from contact, others learned to live without her. In recovery they secretly resent her "returning home" and upsetting the system. How does young daughter Emily give up her "homemaker" role when Mom returns? She has to give up premature power and responsibility. Children often complain that they liked it better when Mom ate because she noticed less of their misdeeds. Even though "Dad yelled a lot," they could get around him, and Mom was really in charge anyway.

FAMILY MESSAGE CENTER

Ralph had alcoholic parents and felt badly about not being able to help them. He married obese Katherine and tried to help her.

Ralph and their seventeen-year-old son Bernard, came to family group therapy. Their first night in family group was early in the mother's recovery. The father started contact by yelling at his son, "Your mom is upset and feels like you are ignoring her." They conversed about this for a few minutes while Katherine watched silently. I asked why Katherine could not tell her son this directly. Ralph had been caretaker for his alcoholic parents and showed his value by being in the middle of family interaction. Mother had early on given over most of her power to him. Thus, he could feel "of value" and she could secretly eat.

I asked her to address her son directly. Katherine began accusing her son of "never paying any attention" to her, always "self-centered," etc. She really needed something from this boy. Rather than ask directly, she had developed a style familiar in addicted families. She began "blaming." She would rather accuse him than share her needs with him.

In the family group session, we asked Katherine to try to find another way to get her needs met.

Therapist: "After all, Katherine, there is something you *want* from this boy. Let's see if you can go at it in a way to get your own needs met."

At this point, Katherine began to cry. Through her tears, she said, "I am so scared that you are angry at me because I need this help. I am afraid you are saying I am a fool and why wasn't I strong enough to handle this on my own."

Instead of judging, Bernard leaned over and hugged her closely. "No Mom. I'm really glad you are finally asking for some help. It's clear you've really been trying on your own, but not getting results. I'll support you in any way I can."

They hugged silently while Katherine sobbed. Dad tried to intervene. He needed to break up some of the closeness so he could feel important again. I reassured him of what a good father he was, and that his best effort would be to let them work it out alone. In this particular family situation, Mother was a secret eater. At first, they all said no one has been affected by the eating. Dad voiced a common refrain, "She eats like a bird." It wasn't her eating that needed review, it was their relating. In this family, Mom was anesthetized. This father and son fought out her grievances. She was never expected to stand up for herself. The two males were kept distant by this.

In recovery, she and her son fight their own battles directly. Now the men can have their own separate relationship. Mom and Dad can also get closer. They don't complain about Bernard so much. They find other things to talk about. If Mom has complaints, she goes directly to the source.

Katherine became very assertive with both her husband and son. When Ralph tried to talk for her, she'd remind him, "Don't speak for me, I can take care of myself." As he stopped being the disciplinarian in the family, he and his son got closer. They even allied with grievances against Mom! Katherine began confronting her husband directly rather than demurely sending her son in. This produced a more conflicted marital relationship for a while, but also a renewed sexual appetite from both partners. As her weight dropped and her insecurities lessened, Katherine felt a new interest in sex and love for her husband. She took Ralph to bed instead of her chocolates.

PLEASE MOM, "I DON'T WANNA GO"

Elvira found that her mom, Vanessa, had built an entire identity around being a mother. Jim and Vanessa Ferguson married because both were graduating college and it seemed the thing to do. Vanessa had majored in home economics and knew her calling was mothering. Relating with Jim was not a priority in her life; she saw him as an instrument on her way to her higher calling: mothering. Even after Elvira moved away to college, the high point of her mother's life was the weekly call from the dorm. Elvira remained Mom's confidante and companion; there was nothing Mom and Dad had to talk to each other about. Elvira was so attached to her mom that she never felt like a real person on her own. Elvira found the only way to be truly alone and independent was after vomiting. Exhausted and spent, she found that a euphoric separateness came over her.

Mother and daughter both enjoyed their relationship tremendously and there seemed no good reason to create distance. The reason emerged when Elvira learned she knew no way to feel like she was living her own life. In recovery she found her mom needed children, but she herself needed to grow up and be her own adult. Her mom saw how much she wanted to be a better mother than *her* mother had been, so she was extremely attached to Elvira. Each was fulfilling someone else's program and had to find an identity that did not involve motherhood. Then Elvira could feel confident to grow up and leave home. Her mother didn't need her to be the child any more. Mom had to give up her caretaker role.

Much has been written about the conflict today's women encounter in forsaking the ideals and expectations of their mothers. In deciding to pursue money, property, and prestige with success in a man's world, daughters are sometimes deciding not to follow some of their mothers' models. This presents some problems when some moms take this as a rejection. There seems to be no way to be true to self *and* loving to Mom. The conflict comes out over the plate or the toilet bowl.

Elvira and her mother had to find a way to say goodbye with love. They needed to cry together; separation is scary and change is disrupting. However, with eating disorders, if we don't take a stand to weather the change, we revert to the old behavior. Vanessa and her daughter were able to cry together. They both found they needed the separation despite the pain of loss. Elvira is beginning to live her own life. She doesn't vomit anymore.

"WE'VE ONLY JUST BEGUN"

How poignant that we will close this chapter quoting a song title Karen Carpenter made famous. Karen died of her eating disorder, anorexia nervosa, even though many protested that "it wasn't anorexia, it was a heart attack." Karen had just regained twenty-five pounds coming out of anorexia with induced medications and her heart could not stand the strain. Karen, though loved by millions of fans, could not find a way to get her neediness filled. Her personal relationships were unsatisfying, and she suffered an E-D's loneliness in the midst of a crowd. Actually, we do die of heart failure, as we die of the inability to find a way to get our hearts filled. Again, the message is, learn to "relate to recover."

THE WEIGH OUT

Chapter Five

Accept That It's Difficult

Now that you both see how you got here, you are at the starting gate to recovery. You will have to face living with a lifelong chronic illness, with personality change as the only reprieve. To give up the love affair with food, you will learn new ways to love and be loved by people. It seems easier to remain judgmental and tease yourself with so called "willpower" and "firm resolve." The rationale to remain aloof and judgmental rather than turning to others seems to have validity. You have been disappointed by other people so often. You chose the secure comfort of food over the unpredictable comfort of other people. Battered and disillusioned, you really can't raise your hopes any more. Hope itself is threatening.

An aged skid row alcoholic I treated growled in group, "I'm John and I'm *no* alcoholic! I'm a *drunk!*" He didn't want to acknowledge having an illness, but instead wanted to judge himself. He later came to realize that derogatory name-calling could keep him drinking, but once he confessed to being an alcoholic, he would see possibilities for help in doing something about it. The recognition leads to recovery.

That same awareness is vital to an E-D's recovery. You must accept that you are different and have different struggles with food. Every normally neurotic American is into dieting. Monday through Friday and alternate weekends, right? That is not your situation. You have an *obsession* with food. It dominates and rules your life. You already addressed the evolution of this obsession to its chronic stage. Now is the moment to admit you can no longer play around with this substance casually. You obviously won't stop eating altogether; but your old obsessive relationship with food has to go.

It isn't easy to admit you are sick. In fact, it is the hardest thing you will ever do. You will have to admit this over and over again. You have surely felt this way before, even if only for a fleeting moment. Then you quickly and conveniently forgot how bad things were.

Really negotiating a lasting recovery involves a constant and deep acceptance of the seriousness of this affliction. This is not easy for you or those who love you. It is especially difficult without the comfort of excess food. Let's begin now to accept the fact that you have spent a lifetime being powerless over food. All of your previous attempts at control have landed you right in this spot now.

ACCEPTING POWERLESSNESS

"Yes, it is that bad . . . and without help it will get worse!" By picking up this book, you took the first essential step to recovery. You already leafed through most of the quickie books and easier, softer ways and found them to be anything but.

The old line goes: There's good news and there's bad news! So, first the bad news. Every E-D must face the fact that they are suffering from a lifelong illness. This illness requires extreme measures to overcome. Recovery from compulsive overeating is difficult; as we said, the most difficult thing you will ever have to do.

Now, the good news. Just because it is difficult doesn't make it impossible. And, as soon as you accept that recovery is difficult— once you understand the disease and the necessity for dramatic change, recovery is no longer so difficult. Amazing as it may seem, saying "We know how hard it is" makes it easier. No matter how many doctors handed you 1200 calorie diets across big brown desks, not one of them has ever said, "I know how hard this is to follow." You were just handed a piece of paper with an implied expectation that you certainly should follow directions. But, if you could have followed those directions, YOU WOULDN'T HAVE BEEN IN THAT OFFICE IN THE FIRST PLACE. You already know what to do. The difficulty is trying to do it alone. I have personally tried all my life to control myself, and I can't. It's embarrassing but true.

It is not easy to reach this stage of profound acceptance. I'm sure you have probably come close before, or you wouldn't be here now, and you probably felt sure you could mobilize all your willpower and fight for as long as you needed to. You got a goal weight and a goal day and clenched your fists to begin. The problem was in assuming that the mobilization would only be needed for a week, a month, a *year* at the very most. We get this idea from the false notion that once we have handled our weight, we have handled our problem. This is not true! Despite your white knuckle resolve, you ended up here. So who wants to face this? Instead:

- We want to believe that all that's wrong with us is a weight problem.
- We refuse to be on a diet for the rest of our lives.
- We promise ourselves, "When I get thin, I'll never, ever gain weight again."

What we end up with are the reasons for failure rather than the results of success. For lasting recovery you will have to buy the idea that you suffer from a lifelong, chronic illness. This must be considered in *all* matters at *all* times. You cannot put it on the back burner and forget it, as much as you might like to. This illness permeated life's every moment. Think about it, how many of your waking hours are spent obsessing about what you will or will not eat, wear or not wear, achieve or not achieve? You must make *recovery* permeate your life as much as the suffering used to. Instead of living a dress rehearsal, you must begin today accepting life where you are now and who you are now. This is not a drill. This is it!

In this chapter you will see where you are on the road to acceptance. The stages are fluid. You may jump back and forth, and could be in two or three stages at once. By the end of the chapter, you will find where you are on the road and identify your own major coping mechanism. Let's begin.

THE ROAD TO ACCEPTANCE

You are being asked to recognize the seriousness of this disease, and the uselessness of simple half measures. I learned this through my own self-observation as well as from sessions with patients who minimized the seriousness of this illness. Later, when I read Dr. Elizabeth Kubler-Ross' description of her work with patients facing imminent death, I was immediately struck by similarities. Her dying patients traveled five distinct stages to reach acceptance: *denial, anger, bargaining, depression,* and finally, *acceptance.* In *On Death and Dying,* Dr. Kubler-Ross concludes that her patients are actually accepting their powerlessness over a force which will soon dominate, and ultimately destroy, their very lives. I saw that other patients traveled these same five stages in accepting any serious illness. This holds true for an overeater, alcoholic, blind man, paraplegic, quadriplegic, or even just an average American. The issue for each is that life has dealt a hand they did not expect or appreciate, but one they would ultimately have to accept.

You do not have to accept this all at once, nor do you even have to feel accepting all the time. "The only way out is through!" states Fritz Perls, father of Gestalt therapy. As Dr. Perls puts it, "Once we accept fully and completely exactly who and what we are, we have then given up the struggle to 'be someone else.' " In accepting ourselves, we automatically become someone else. In other words, we move from being a self-hater—a person who says, "I should be different"—to a person who echoes Popeye the sailor and says, "I am what I am and that's all what I am."

SELF-ACCEPTANCE

Are you really ready for self-acceptance? Can you take the necessary steps to accept where you are right now as the best of all possible worlds? Even if you don't like it can you accept that it must be the correct, consequence of your whole life to this point? Can you accept that where you are is where you should be? You may have to face a lot. See how much of the following you can buy:

- Your best friend, food, has turned on you.
- You have tried everything already and ended up right here.
- Your obsession with food fits right in with how you have been living your life.
- No guru out there is going to fix it for you.
- It's got the best of you.

When Dr. Kubler-Ross first approached a hospital to counsel the dying patients, she asked the staff where they were kept. Agitated and fearful nurses told her, "Oh, no one dies here."

This occured in hospitals with elaborate procedures for the care of dying patients and definite courses of action taken once a patient died. The hospitals had their own morgue and even separate driveways for hearses. Still, the answer she received from the staff of more than one hospital was, "Oh, no one dies here."

This is denial in its most blatant form. Thus, Dr. Kubler-Ross' first task was confronting the denial system. The denial we see in eating disorders is no less blatant and no less difficult to confront. Sufferers who admit they have problems won't accept a lifelong chronic illness. Facing the severity of the disease is just as hard as accepting death.

In facing compulsive eating, the denial stage is probably the most prevalent and definitely the deadliest. You deny the harsh reality of having a chronic and often terminal illness. You desperately want to believe you really have a minor ailment which you will soon treat—"as soon as I'm ready." You deny that the illness is affecting every area of your life and that its arrest will require major life changes. "I know I can diet whenever I want to," you say. "I'll start tomorrow, or next Monday." How many years has that gone on? You would like this to be a simple project that won't require too much effort or too much disruption in your lifestyle. To think like that is to remain self-deluded; believing that the whole thing is "no big deal, I can handle it myself." You don't recognize how pervasive denial has become.

Here is another aspect of denial which is often reinforced by well-meaning codependents. "All you need is a little more willpower," they exclaim. This only adds guilt and self-loathing. The truth is, lack of willpower is not a characteristic of E-Ds. On the contrary, most have an abundance of determination and willpower. You often become the best workers in misguided attempts to make up for the food obsession. You are often known as "really good friends," always there in time of need. You typically exhibit a great deal of power and strength. All of which, of course, does nothing for your lifelong, terminal illness. At this point it should be obvious that *willpower has absolutely nothing to do with this illness!*

Yet, denial does not stop even here. Many of you try wearing bright clothing and jewelry or eye-catching hairdos, hoping that no one will notice the fat. But surely, it seems you must be able to see the enormity of your flesh! How can you deny so obvious a problem? Quite easily, and here's how. E-Ds, whether you are fat or thin, have no realistic sense of your own body image. You have spent many years with a fluid body configuration. One year you wore size twelve all summer and then the next year size 24 seems snug. It seems reasonable to think that "the dryer is shrinking my clothes." Most of you put on and take off weight so fast that you amass great poundage without even noticing. Not seeing realistically is a way to continue the weight gain/loss cycle.

You have gained and lost thousands of pounds throughout your life, so you assume this is normal for all folks. You have spent countless mornings paying homage to a flat, spring-driven contraption you have made into a god—the great god called The Scale. Surely this god won't let you down. Yet, even this god cannot conquer denial!

Take the case of Patricia. She is an attractive and intelligent businesswoman with a definite image of herself and what her poundage should be. She knew when she was overweight, and she was intellectually very clear about the top weight she would never surpass. Her weight fluctuated between 150–180 pounds. This was her "hovering weight," the numbers around which she could hover. If the Great Scale God reported these figures, all was still right with her world. After each bout with a newly published diet, or before a social event where dress size was the goal and fasting the method, Patricia expected to weigh in at about 150 pounds. Conversely, between Thanksgiving and New Year's, or after a vacation trip, she expected to weigh close to 180. This was somewhat distasteful, albeit predictable, understandable, and acceptable. It fit in with her self-concept and what she expected out of life. Patricia knew that if she ever hit 181, an alarm bell would immediately send her to pills or fat farms. Her self-image remained intact and all was right with the world, because she weighed no more than 180 pounds. Then something happened.

Unexpected professional reverses drove Patricia into seeking solace with even more excess food. Bingeing helped her work later hours, trying to recoup her losses. Her food consumption continued unchecked. Patricia did not find time to get on a scale for three months. This is not unusual. It is quite common for denial systems to help misplace scales, calorie counters, or tight-fitting clothing. Patricia forged on, oblivious to everything.

Then, when the business crisis was finally over and Patricia once more found her bathroom scale, she weighed 202 pounds! Impossible! This figure would not register with her image of who she was. Denial sprang up like a demon to keep Patricia's self-image intact. "There must be some mechanical error," it crooned to her. Patricia's answer was quite simple—she threw away the scale. Absurd? Maybe. Yet this is not uncommon for E-Ds. Many have not weighed themselves for years. First the scale is worshipped, then renounced. This is denial.

Patricia must first weigh in and face the scale. She must face reality and smash denial. She must take a look at how, using excessive work pressures as the excuse, she keeps bingeing. In order to say no to excess food, she may have to say no to some of the work assignments. She would prefer to just diet rather than face having to make changes in her daily lifestyle. She needs to risk to recover.

In the same way that you deny physical reality, you deny psychological reality. Your life is filled with secrets you keep from yourself and others. You have kept your eating behavior secret, and lived in a private emotional hell. You rarely tell people how you feel. This holds true for the "people pleaser" who is always sweet and charming, as well as for the brash confrontive "tough guy" who never seems to experience a weak moment. Both of these stereotyped images, common to overeaters, deny the existence of their opposites. You must face the undeniable fact that we are as sick as we are secret. Without her food, the "jolly old fat lady" may uncover the bitch she's been suppressing, and the "tough survivor" may have to spend some time falling apart.

Marnie was jolly, competent, and already successfully losing weight when I confronted her denial system.

"But I've just lost 120 pounds! Why would I need help?" Marnie seemed astonished that I had approached her about becoming a patient in treatment. She weighed over 600 pounds! She found breathing difficult. Her chest was so heavy her lungs were unable to expand, and so she suffered frequent dizziness from lack of oxygen. She had heard my lecture to a community group about the opening of a new HOPE Unit dedicated to Helping Overeaters through People and Education. She approached me later to ask if we had a job opening, mentioning she was an excellent secretary. I smiled and took her number, agreeing to call her the following week. I felt we

both understood that she was really approaching me for professional help, not employment.

I was surprised when she again mentioned her secretarial skills at our meeting. Her own personal denial system was so effective that it had walled her off from reality entirely. There is nothing else that adequately explains why a 600-pound woman would deny a need for help. She did indeed want to overcome her lifelong, chronic problem, but wouldn't admit she'd need help. She was terrified at the prospect of facing the full dimensions of the problem. She had indeed lost a great deal of weight already and wanted to believe she could make it on her own. Denial sings, "I can do it myself." In later therapy, we discovered that the "120 pounds" she claimed to have lost was actually a figure she had made up. Since it had been impossible to weigh her, no one really knew. She also admitted that the lost weight was returning; her muumuus were getting tighter. Weighing more than can be recorded on a scale has a certain element of personal security—poundage can come and go without record. It is possible to continue to deny the problem without definite evidence. Chronically obese all her life, a weight swing of 20 or 30 pounds in 48 hours was "normal" for someone like Marnie.

At our first meeting, we sat down with a counselor to discuss why she had come to the hospital. She again quickly pointed out her office managerial skills. She convinced the counselor that she was very adept at controlling and managing office situations, but her body attested to her inadequate *self*-control. We gently directed the conversation away from office proficiency and toward psychological pain. The counselor, a compulsive overeater in recovery, told of maintaining a weight loss of over 100 pounds, and that she remembered her own attempts to show off at work so that no one would notice she was fat. That helped melt Marnie's denial system and at last she opened up. She admitted to hoping she could get some help by working there. Later she saw how she was hoping to "bootleg" therapy and gain help by working with us rather than painfully admitting her own desperate neediness. She wanted to help others as a way of staying in denial. It can't happen through osmosis. With addictive disorders, an essential ingredient for success is that you face your own denial and admit within your own heart a personal need for help. The help may be professional, but doesn't have to

be. Families and friends can help, or new friends in Overeaters Anonymous can help. To recover, you have to become vulnerable and ask before anyone else can have an effect.

CODEPENDENTS ALSO DENY

The same hopes of clearing it up "next Monday," or minimizing the importance of the obsession happens for codependents, also. In fact, many times the codependent is in even more denial than the E-D. The codependent denies the seriousness by pretending it will "clear up" soon. This denial helps the E-D keep bingeing. Here, for example, is a common scenario between E-Ds and codependents.

> E-D: Dear, do you think I'm as fat as that lady over there?
> Codependent: Oh, I don't know. It's really hard to tell.
> E-D: Well, please take a look. I just want to know the truth.
> Codependent: Well, er, no, you're not. I think she's fatter than you.
> E-D: Thanks, I really wanted to know.

I can't recall ever hearing such an interchange with the codependent answering, "Well, truthfully, you are actually much fatter than that lady." When the E-D knows she will hear that answer, she will not ask. She only asks when she knows someone will help her maintain denial.

Another way codependents help in denial is when they assume a punitive parent role with the E-D. In this case, they are telling the truth, "You are fat," but they do it in a way that minimizes how difficult recovery is. This is where they deny the seriousness of the project by cajoling or manipulating with hints of diets or controlling the E-D's food. They may yell and threaten, all as a way to keep believing willpower will fix it.

> Codependent: Why don't you do something about your weight?
> E-D: I'm really trying. I want to do it for *you.*
> Codependent: Bull! You don't care about me.
> E-D: Yes I do. I want you to be proud of me.

Codependent: Sure! If you really loved me, you'd take care of it.

E-D: I can't help it. I want to, but can't.

Codependent: I don't believe you. In fact, if you don't get it together I'm going to leave you!

In this exchange, the codependent has become punitive as a result of hurt and disappointment. The codependent is denying that the E-D is actually trying but still failing. You don't want to believe them and you are powerless. You take it personally with the "if you loved me" approach. The E-D's problem is not a slap in the face to you. The E-D is not doing it to you. They're doing it because they are sick. Denying that this is an illness keeps us hammering away at symptoms rather than causes.

Many suffer with other lifelong, chronic illnesses such as alcoholism, diabetes, and tuberculosis. A symptom of untreated alcoholism is that people must drink. A symptom of tuberculosis is that people must cough. A symptom of an eating disorder is that people must eat compulsively. We do not approach the tubercular patient and say, "If you loved me, you'd stop coughing." Why do we think stopping eating has anything to do with love?

A healthier response is, "Dear, I am very happy you asked me for my opinion. I know you love me, but hurt yourself. I have noticed you suffering about your weight; that you feel guilty and scared. It seems like you really are motivated and trying. I can offer you my love and support if you are willing to get help. I really don't think you can keep tackling this thing alone. I also see that I can't help you."

How the E-D gets help, then, is none of your business. He or she may seek hospital treatment, work in partnership with a friend, join a diet club, or, as I suggest, attend Overeaters Anonymous. In any event, your position is to be supportive. Strange as it may seem, you can't include yourself directly in the helping system. You will need your own help in letting him or her quit alone.

EXERCISE: DEALING WITH DENIAL

Check the following statements you have said or thought in the past year:

I can't find my scale. _____

I'm still within "hovering weight." _____

My hairdo gives me height. _____

This food in my mouth has nothing to do with the fat on my body. _____

The scale is broken. _____

The dryer is shrinking my clothes. _____

It is a minor ailment that will clear up as soon as I am ready. _____

I can go on a diet and lose weight whenever I want to. _____

I'm going to start tomorrow or next Monday. _____

This is a simple project and won't really require too much effort or disruption in my life. _____

This is no big deal. I can handle it myself. _____

All I need is willpower. _____

I am so accomplished in other areas, I should be able to do this easily. _____

It's not my fault; who wouldn't eat with a husband, wife, mother, father like mine? _____

I have to eat this way to maintain my job. _____

I don't really eat very much at all. I eat like a bird. _____

I am really not my body; I am really something else. _____

I can lose weight as easily as I gained it. _____

I like "slenderizing" clothes. _____

I guess it is slight water retention. _____

If you recall thinking any of the foregoing three or more times last year, denial may be your major coping mechanism. You probably avoid acceptance by staying in the denial stage.

I'M MAD AS HELL

"Why me? It's just not fair!" Of course, you're right. "Look at that skinny thing over there; she eats anything she wants and never gains a pound. Why was I dealt this rotten hand? Why must I live so stringently? Why am I so deprived?" The lament goes on.

As an E-D, whether male or female, you are angry at God, fate, and a society dictating a body standard that borders on painfully thin. You are angry at the kid at the beach yelling, "Hey, Mom, look at the fat lady over there," or "Gee, look how fat that man is."

You are mad for all the lost years, the proms not attended, the outings refused. Anger is probably the most prevalent underlying emotion an E-D knows, yet it is also the hardest to express. You have spent so many years practicing the art of "people pleasing" so you could fit in despite repulsive looks. You overcompensate so no one will notice the fat by being overachievers and wonderfully helpful friends. However, buried many layers deep, you are very, very angry.

Suppressed anger must be brought to the surface. It would be unrealistic to expect someone who has spent a lifetime in self-abuse, to say nothing of abuse from others, to immediately feel serene, self-satisfied and content. You have to vent anger first. Usually, very little work is required for this anger to emerge. When you stop eating compulsively, anger automatically erupts within days. These raging feelings have been boiling under the surface, and only kept under control by the sedation of food. Have you noticed how irritating everyone at home becomes the day you start a new diet? Is it them or you?

Anger should not just be allowed, but actually promoted and encouraged. Codependents, take cover! The anger is often vented against those nearest and dearest, and especially those trying to help. You see, you know your best friend, food, is being taken away. Whoever is close seems to be the one who is taking it away. You have to strike out. There is absolutely no reason you should like the idea of having a chronic illness, or facing life without comfort from food. You don't know any other way to get comfort yet. You are still scared of people. You bet you feel threatened and angry!

As a codependent, if you want to stay around, you will need to develop a fairly thick skin at this point. The E-D will need to express all kinds of rage. You must decide if you want to be the one to listen, or if you want to suggest they turn to others instead. You don't have to be the garbage can. In ancient Rome, when a messenger brought bad news, his tongue was cut out. Romans went directly to the source of the information. That is exactly what an E-D feels like doing to anyone who tries to help them. They will be striking out blindly as they face how hard it is. You don't have to be the one to bear the brunt of these tidings. The anger is not necessarily at you. If you step out of the way, the E-D will find others who can help in sorting out where all the rage belongs.

The anger must be expressed or it will only be drowned again with food abuse. BE ANGRY NOW AND THINNER LATER. The codependent's choice is, take it on or get out of the way.

EXERCISE: AGITATING ANGER

Check the phrases you have said or thought in the past year.

It's really not fair!	_____
Who says I can't eat that?	_____
How the hell can you help me?	_____
You are an incompetent helper!	_____
That skinny bitch can eat whatever she wants.	_____
Clothes are made to rip. Cheap!	_____
They're fanatic in showing off bodies.	_____
I know they're out to get me.	_____

Add whatever angry responses you've noticed from yourself. (Since so many are hidden anger blockers, much of your anger was masked while you smiled and kept still.)

Don't worry if you don't feel angry now. All you have to do is cut down the eating and believe me, it will emerge! It's been drowned by food and is just waiting to get out.

I have seen one patient who did not go through this angry irritation stage. I was concerned and uneasy about her treatment. She remained pleasant and serene. She never got irritated about anything. It didn't fit! Eventually she cleared up the confusion. She admitted in group therapy that she had been secretly stealing food out of the refrigerator late at night. Her rage had been kept in check through well-practiced and familiar means—food.

Vomiting is often a way to express rage that seems inappropriate. This was certainly true for fourteen-year-old Cindy, who vomited ten times a day rather than talk with her family about their excessive secrecy and anger with each other. Cindy became the family symptom as she sought help to stop vomiting.

Her father, Mel, a middle manager with a west coast firm, enjoys a prominent position and is highly respected. Attractive and stately, although somewhat pudgy, he looks appropriate for his years and position. He and Janelle had married when both were developing careers, and she became his able companion up the corporate ladder. Her alcoholic parents had separated when she was nine months old and she grew up living out her mother's worries about abandonment and financial insecurity. She resolved she would marry success and make it happen. She would also work to cheer up her somewhat stodgy husband and make him happy. Instead, by the time Cindy was negotiating her adolescence, Mel and Janelle were approaching divorce. No one talked, but all raged within.

Janelle was wraith-like thin. Her drawn face framed piercing eyes, and her body contorted rigidly, signalling the pent-up emotions within. Sitting motionless was her way to mask the rage she felt, but her right hand would contort into a fist on her lap. Her knuckles were white, and she found it difficult to unclench. She was holding on for dear life.

Cindy accommodated her mother's need to express rage by binge-ing and vomiting. Obsessed with carbohydrates, she also wanted to be as thin as her mother. She didn't know how to eat away at herself from inside as Janelle did. (Janelle had previously been treated for ulcers and colitis, physical responses to blocked emotion.) Cindy had to juggle a love of food with a desire to be thin. She felt all her mother's feelings and didn't know what to do with them. Vomiting became a workable solution.

When I approached Janelle about the necessity for treating the whole family, she balked. "I am on my way out of this marriage. I don't want to be talked back into it." I didn't know then that Janelle had been saying this for the past nineteen years. Later she explained that she was staying just long enough to "get some financial security" so she wouldn't suffer like her own mother had. (Actually Janelle had already suffered her own mother's pain *and* her own. Cindy would suffer her mother's pain in the same way.)

Mel had been having an affair which caused him extreme guilt and anxiety. His secret relationship with his secretary had been dis-covered and he had vowed to fire her and end it. He later secretly rehired her, hiding that fact from everyone except fourteen-year-old Cindy. He was using Cindy as his confidante, but at her expense. This gave her an unnatural and overly important role in her family.

At a time when she would naturally be working toward separation and independence, she was instead used as the family message center. She was in a double bind for which vomiting proved the only outlet.

As family members became more honest in recovery, secrets came out into the open. Mel talked about his guilt and self-loathing and his desire to do whatever it took to end the family's suffering. He later stopped blaming himself so much and realized that he had not been able to open up in the marriage, but did deserve to get love and support for himself. Janelle later revealed that she knew that the affair had resumed, but was waiting around until she "amassed enough money." She didn't see that this man was not like her father and would make a fair financial settlement in divorce. (They also lived in a "community property" state where assets are legally divided 50–50.) Therefore, Janelle really stayed for other than financial reasons. Cindy was displaced from her job as the family secret bearer. When all cards were out, her vomiting stopped. Dad's secret affair was disclosed, Mom's plans to leave were exposed, and Cindy was refocused to care for herself. Her illness became her first priority. She saw that her parents had their relationship and intrigues long before she was around and it was not her job to worry about them. With that, the parents entered divorce mediation counseling and Cindy got on with the business of growing up. Her parents had to find a more appropriate avenue for their anger with each other rather than routing it through Cindy.

"LET'S MAKE A DEAL"

You will want to maintain some sense of power over this illness. You want to feel in control. You want to change the results without changing what you're doing. But *it can't be done!* You can't keep "the same old me" and gain recovery. Your life must change, then the obsession will follow. Now, no one really wants to hear that, so you will search after easier, softer ways and busy yourself with half measures. That's exactly what dieting is all about. You want to kid yourself that this is purely a physical problem. "It's my glands." "It's low blood sugar—a high protein diet will take care of it." You bargain with the disease and in the process deny how serious it really is.

Similarly, you try to bargain with the time and effort required to recover. "I only want to attend meetings once a week." "I don't see why I should give up my vacation plans just because they happen to fall smack in the middle of a treatment program."

Not only do you want to bargain about how seriously you need to invest in recovery, you also want to bargain about what is needed in terms of personal change. "I'd like to change my relationship with my sister, but I don't want to talk to my mother." Or, "My spouse and I can benefit from this, but there is really no need to involve the children." Or, "I wouldn't want to ask *them* to help me."

In the angry stage you rebelled: "Why me? I don't want this! Give it to someone else." In the bargaining stage, you accept that you have this affliction and that it will not be easy to overcome. *But* . . . you still want to make some attempts on your own. This stage is both comical and devastating. Here is where you try the various diet fads, pills, shots, acupuncture needles, meditation, hypnosis, protein drinks, health foods, etc., etc., etc. All of these are short-run pretentions. Each new plan helps continue the delusion. You want to believe in the myth of self-sufficiency while dying inside. Many continue on with the bargaining and undergo none of the major relationship changes that could bring a lifelong, stable recovery.

Conversely, some try changing relationships without giving up the obsessive relationships with food. Many of my therapist friends are constantly involved in helping others in order to hide their own neediness, and continue eating compulsively. They go to weekend workshops and retreats and learn psychological interpretations, meditations, Sufi dancing, and Reichian explosions—all the while bingeing on nuts, fruits, and "healthy" grains. Some binge for weeks and then seclude themselves in health farms for a few days of fasting, only to begin again. They are pretending that personal insight alone can lead to cure. They do this bargaining while still bingeing. Insight without abstinence is not enough. Also, abstinence without insight is not enough. It is a physical *and* psychological illness. You can't treat one half and not the other. It's a package deal!

Included in the bargaining phase are the myriad treatment approaches which avoid looking at the basic underlying personality structure and instead focus solely on the physical. These include all shots and pills, diet clubs, gyms and sanitariums, health spas and fat farms, surgical procedures, shock treatments, nutritional counseling, and bibliotherapy (the many and varied volumes E-Ds purchase and discard; they all told us it would be easy).

Essentially, bargaining addresses isolated aspects of your life. You compartmentalize yourself and assume an unrealistic power of the mind over the body or vice versa. These approaches fail to integrate the mind, body, and spirit. You will need to address all aspects of the illness to gain lasting recovery. Most of these other methods promote the idea that recovery is time-limited, and that you can undergo a certain "treatment" and thus achieve cure. You want to believe you can do something and be finished once and for all. You see it as a kind of exorcism. "Such a deal" has been the lifelong wish of every compulsive eater, and it only serves to keep you fat.

Morris was just such a bargainer. He was tall, blond, and gigantic! He was thirty years old and weighed 594 pounds. As he entered the lecture hall where I was speaking, a number of people moved aside. His size alone intimidated most. He was accustomed to people getting out of his way and being somewhat fearful around him. Later, in recovery, he admitted this was a puzzle to him, as he felt so "tiny inside." When he eventually stopped eating compulsively, he felt like a little boy, not the giant he had become. Everyone else viewed him as big and tough, so he acted out the part for his audience.

No seat in the auditorium was big enough, so he slouched against the back wall to listen. Before I finished with introductory remarks, his questions boomed loudly from the back of the room. "Why do you talk about this being an illness? Don't you think that's discouraging to people?" As I tried to explain that accepting it as difficult made it easier, in a sense, Morris boomed again, "Well, isn't it a matter of willpower, and if a person really wants to, they can?"

I asked him if he could answer that based on his own experience. He was quick to reply, "I've had a weight problem for years, but I've never really tried to diet. My weight has not really been a problem for me. I am energetic and personable; my friends call me the life of the party. I don't see why you refer to overweight people as sick." At this point, others in the audience asked Morris to be quiet and allow the lecture to continue. I was, admittedly, intimidated, but went on.

Morris remained quiet for the rest of the hour. Later, when

others approached the podium to ask personal questions, Morris disappeared out the side door.

A week later he called. With no greeting and no mention of his name, he blurted out, "I want to find out more of what you're about."

"In what way?" I asked.

"What kind of treatment are you suggesting?"

At this point, I recognized the gruff voice and asked for his name. "You don't need to know that yet. I want to know first if you have anything to offer that could interest me."

"Didn't you say you had never tried to diet and never seen your weight as a problem?" I replied.

"I still don't see it as a problem and really don't think I need help. It's just that the coach of my basketball team is bugging me." I was shocked to discover that a man of this grotesque size was capable of playing basketball. Imagine what he might have weighed without such strenuous sports activities! I proceeded to outline a typical regimen undertaken by most successful patients. This included attendance at group therapy sessions three nights each week. "Well, that is ridiculous. I can't make that kind of commitment. I have my basketball practice. I'm certainly not going to give that up. I know the coach wouldn't want that." He thanked me and hung up.

It was two months before he called again. "The coach is becoming a real pain in the ass!" I knew right away who it was and didn't ask his name this time. "So maybe, I could get involved with your program if I could come once a week and still make practice regularly."

"I'm sorry," I said. "We've found that this particular plan works best for the greatest number of people and I think you deserve the benefit of full treatment." I have found that if we keep everyone committed to the same plan, they all usually do well. The special cases where exceptions are made produce more complications and mistakes. Surgical teams in most major hospitals can attest to this. When they admit a doctor or doctor's wife for any type of surgical procedure, the incidence of complication is statistically higher. Instead of treating them like a routine case, everyone works to put in special effort to insure the finest quality care. What often happens is overzealousness, which leads to incompetence, and they end up with more problems. As I tried to explain this to Morris, he hung up again.

His next call came within the month. As I answered the phone, he began, "Surely you can understand that a person's physical activity is important for their emotional and physical well-being. Don't you believe in exercise for healthy bodies?"

"Sure I do," I replied, "but your exercising has not really helped you cut down on compulsive eating."

"How do you know how I eat? That's really none of your business."

"I do know that for anyone to get as big as you are, even while playing basketball, they certainly have to pack in a lot of food. Your exercising may be serving as a perfect excuse to keep you binge-ing."

He hung up. I didn't hear from him for three more months. When he called again, he sounded forlorn. The fight was out of his voice. The hurt was there. "I've really been trying to handle this thing on my own. I seem to go along fine for a week or more, but then end up running from one 7–11 store to another. My apartment is strewn with straws and wrappers. There's a three foot pile of garbage around my bed."

I responded with, "Sounds like your experience is common to many of us. The more we try to control it, the more it dominates our lives. I'm really happy you are calling. Could you tell me your name?"

At that point he told me his name was Morris. Then he quickly pointed out that even if others had done as he had, his case was "quite different." He wanted me to know that his being a young and brilliant engineer coupled with his athletic ability made his situation special. He tried to convince me, "Since I am very intelligent, I pick up information and learn much more rapidly than most people. Don't you think I could get along with coming to therapy less often than others?" His tone had turned from hostile to pleading, but I still had to say no.

"I assure you I am giving you the best recommendation I can, based on my own professional experience. Why don't you give yourself the full chance you deserve and jump into recovery with both feet?"

His curt response was, "You won't be hearing from me again!"

And he slammed down the phone. Following the progression, you can see how Morris moved from denial that he even had a problem to bargaining with the schedule recommended for his recovery, and into anger at me for bringing the possibility of help to him in the first place.

Morris' negotiations with me to help him get away with doing less are all part of the bargaining stage. We call his "specialness" position "terminal uniqueness."

TERMINAL UNIQUENESS

"If the other guy had to pay a dime for it, let me pay a nickel."
"My case is different."
"I need special handling."
"I'm not as bad as all that."
"Give me a good deal."
"Nobody gets the better of me."
"I'm not a schmuck like everybody else."

Unfortunately, the eating disorder brings everyone to their knees in having to face human fallibility. No one is "better than" or "less than" anyone else, and we're all in the human race together. Morris was using basketball as a way to set himself apart from others. His ego ran rampant across the basketball court, but his need for human closeness was submerged in his bed with a television set and a bag of Oreo cookies.

Four months later, Morris was kicked off the team. He had gained twenty more pounds. For Morris, the basketball coach had been his codependent. The coach had tried to get Morris to accept help, but didn't feel secure enough to be forceful about it. The coach had a lot to gain from Morris' skill on the court. Morris was his star player. Morris ran harder and pushed himself more than anyone on the team. His spirit and drive motivated the other players. The coach was willing to keep Morris, even fat, rather than risk losing him completely. However, when the twenty extra pounds came on, the coach was terrorized every time he watched his star player move down the court. Morris became so red and bloated that a heart attack looked imminent. The coach had no choice, and Morris' bargaining prove expensive.

Morris never did say "I need help" out loud. When he called

he simply said, "This is Morris. Where do I sign?" In his case, he had to lose the very thing he was bargaining to preserve before he was willing to commit himself to recovery. Sometimes, the thing we are absolutely, resolutely, unwilling to give up becomes the very thing we have to let go. That applies whether we are striking the bargain for basketball, homes, jobs, husbands, wives, cars, or children. We have to contemplate that we'll *lose to win*.

Morris ultimately recovered much more than he gave up. He was back on the team within three months. He has let go of over three hundred pounds. He's newly married and expecting a baby. He still plays basketball, but he can take it or leave it. It doesn't own him. He doesn't need it to fulfill ego needs to overcompensate for his physical deformity. People don't move aside when he enters a room. In fact, he's become so warm and cuddly that many reach out to him with hugs. What a deal!

EXERCISE: BARGAIN POOR

Check the statements you have said or thought during the past year.

I will diet Monday through Friday, but binge on weekends. _____

I will change to eating only at meal times and not in between. _____

I will eat smaller portions all day long. _____

I will only eat in the kitchen. _____

I will spend $300 for this exercise gym. _____

I will go to a health spa for two weeks. _____

I will buy an exercycle. _____

I will go to a steam bath. _____

I will wear sweatsuits. _____

I will go for cellulite therapy. _____

I will have an intestinal bypass operation. _____

I will have a stomach staple. _____

I will take diet pills. _____

Add in some more of your own "unique" bargains.

_____ _____

_____ _____

_____ _____

_____ _____

IT'S OKAY TO FEEL BAD

American society frowns on feeling bad about anything. "Keep a stiff upper lip," "Let a smile be your umbrella," "Oh, you're just feeling sorry for yourself." And yet, despite all the cultural taboos, it is essential that the E-D *feel* the pain and hopelessness of the condition. You must face the tragedy of the illness and experience mourning and loss. You must give up the lifelong delusion that you don't have a problem. It will make you sad. You must face the fact that life is not a dress rehearsal, but that "this is it and it stinks." It won't get better on its own. Recovery won't be easy. In fact, it will be the hardest thing you've ever undertaken. All other life projects will pale in comparison.

The past was undertaken with the comfort of a lifelong friend and faithful companion—food. Now you will face losing this friendship. You must look at the wasted teenage years and all the other time damaged by this illness. Only by facing these things can you muster the energy to recover.

Seeing the lifelong wish for easy answers shattered invariably results in deep depression and mourning; mourning the loss of a dream, mourning the hope that the easy thin life is right around the corner. Every E-D has offered up the secret prayer: "God, let me make it this time and I'll never be fat again," only to face the despair of another weight gain later. To recover you must mourn the loss of a simple cure.

Most have lived in a dress rehearsal, preparing for that ever elusive time "when I get thin." Without drastic measures, without a total life reorganization, you are doomed to repeat the same cyclical patterns. Therefore, to accept recovery, you must first mourn the old way of life!

Noted psychologist Carl Jung said, "There is no birth of consciousness without pain." E-Ds who truly accept recovery must lay old patterns to rest and give birth to a new life. There is pain, and you need to cry. You need to mourn the loss of your comforting food. The relationship, as you knew it, is gone forever. A new relationship with food will take its place.

Codependents are vitally affected in this stage, and, as a codependent, you must "release with love" enough to allow E-Ds to experience their own pain. You may want to try to shelter and protect them. Family members will usually encourage avoidance of pain. You want to offer some diverting activity to keep the E-D's mind off the problem. Even if you were super-judgmental and critical before, you may now become supreme rescuers. Please be aware of what you are doing. You may be trying to soothe your own pain. You are depressed that all your efforts have not succeeded in helping your loved one. You are facing your own powerlessness.

One husband became quite upset when his wife cried in group therapy. His first offer of solace was, "Come on, dear, I'll take you out to dinner and we'll forget about all this." He needs instead to find a way to offer "tough love" and respect the E-D enough to let her cry her own tears.

As a codependent, the best way to help an E-D with depression is by being an example as you face yours. When you see that recovery involves changing relationships, you will anticipate losses for you, as well. You will have your own mourning and depression.

LOSE TO WIN

There are losses for all family members in recovery. You have actually been too close, and will need to develop some breathing space. You will be facing the pain of growing up and leaving home. You will be leaving the security of all you've known and stepping out into a new way of life.

This growing up and leaving home takes a much longer time in the United States than any other culture. This may account for why we are so much more obese than the rest of the world. Primitive tribes negotiate this rite of passage at the onset of puberty. Instead, we remain childlike and emotionally infantile, sometimes until death. It is no accident that eating disorders bloom in adolescence. Perhaps we have not learned effective ways to grow up and leave the nest.

Other animals have a much easier time with this than humans. Perhaps it is because they're willing to suffer the pain of separation. A British television documentary shows well how the natural world negotiates this phenomenon with red foxes in Alaska. The film, "Cry of the Wild," shows a den of red foxes where the mother has died. The father was left to raise the pups. As they approached a year old, it was time for these babies to leave the nest. It was Dad's job to kick them out. This resulted in a knock-down, drag-out fight with blood all over the snow. These young foxes did not want to go. Winter was approaching, snow was falling, and they wanted to stay home. Dad didn't care. "No, you gotta get out," he growled. They fought through the night. Smaller and weaker, by daybreak the babies whimpered away.

The scene was quite sad, especially for Dad, who was left alone in his empty nest. His wife was gone, kids were gone, but it was something he *had* to do. He had a natural instinct to help his children suffer the pain of growth. With no therapy, and little thought, he just did what he had to do.

When winter came, he and they stalked the woods alone. He was sad, but he'd done the right thing. With the spring thaw, all the little pups came back to visit. They returned as totally new entities. They strutted up to the den, proud and separate. The walk was different. They were in a whole new relationship with him. Some brought their new-found mate alongside. It was clear that this was *his* place and they were coming to visit a while and then be on their own way.

Daddy fox had done his kids a favor. He helped them learn about "differentness." He almost had to kill them to teach them, but it was something they had to learn. When they returned, there was mutual respect on both sides. Although it was painful, he helped them each separate and become themselves.

The same pain has to be weathered, especially by mothers and daughters, or you will have to keep amassing flesh to feel grounded and separate. You will have to consider the pain of growing up as an alternative to the pain of your eating disorder.

LOSSES FOR THE CODEPENDENT

Losing Predictable Patterns. Before, it was all quite simple. You knew exactly what to say that would make them mad or quiet them down and they knew the same about you. There are many surprises in store now. Maybe you won't like such a risky business. You might prefer the old system. You used to know how to light up their keyboard. Maybe it was a pile of manure, but you knew what it smelled like. As you mourn the loss of the old predictable response patterns, you can get turned on to the excitement of meeting a "new person" to have a new relationship.

Losing Security.   You once felt secure in the attitude that, "I'm the best thing that ever happened to her. She certainly can't do better." You may find it difficult to be in a relationship where the other person is with you out of choice. Ultimately though, you'll feel more secure later when you see they're still around because they want to be.

Losing a Scapegoat.   It was once quite easy to blame problems on the E-D, but who do you blame now? What if the E-D gets better, but you uncover other problems? It might seem safer to keep the Eating Disorder as the focus of your discontent, but it's not. When you face real problems during recovery, they can heal in the open air rather than festering unattended.

Losing Martyrdom.   No longer can you represent yourself as the one who is "sticking it out" despite all obstacles. You won't get any more praise for endurance. In fact, you may see the E-D praised for abstinence and feel jealous! But, you'll find a way to get your own strokes for yourself. Instead of praise for suffering, you'll be encouraged to go for even more happiness.

Losing a Caretaker Role.   When the E-D takes full responsibility for his or her own recovery, you may feel like your child has been snatched from your arms. Who will you care for now? It's hard to be out of a job. You may want to seek out another, sicker E-D to fix. Don't. Try to face just being happy without fixing anyone.

Losing False Esteem.   Your identity has been closely linked with the E-D. You established your personality based on comparing yourself with someone else. You used to be able to say, "At least I'm better than THAT!" What do you say now? Now you can find out who you really are.

Losing Retribution.   If you truly accept that the E-D behaved in certain ways because of the sickness, then you have to stop blaming. That's a lot to give up. You may want him or her to atone for the past. What do you do with your vengeful feelings?

As a codependent you will also have to accept that you chose to endure and live the way you have. No one is responsible for your past but you. Just like the E-D, you did the best you could with what you knew then. You may want to mourn for some of the time you wasted. You, too, have invested years in wishing and waiting. Now that there is hope of recovery, you may feel safe enough to let the pain out and cry for yourself. You'll cry about who you've become. Like the classic fairy tale, you thought you could turn your E-D into a prince or princess with a kiss. Instead, *you* turned into a FROG!

EXERCISE: DELVE INTO DEPRESSION

Check the statements you have said or thought.

This is hopeless. _____

It seems like I just had to keep eating like that. _____

I can't continue like this. _____

I really screwed up my whole life. _____

We're both failures. _____

I'm afraid you won't need me anymore. _____

I haven't been able to talk to you. _____

We both missed out on a lot. _____

Why didn't we see this sooner? _____

There's no comfort without food. _____

There's no comfort with food. _____

It's not worth it. _____

It's not fair. _____

I'm afraid if I change, people won't like me. _____

Add more of your own:

_____ _____

_____ _____

_____ _____

_____ _____

ACCEPTANCE AT LAST

When depression is allowed, it passes. When it is denied, it festers. It goes underground through use of food and other drugs, and serves to help deaden every other feeling. You need help to weather the depression. You can then move into a meaningful acceptance of the illness. "The only way *out* is *through.*"

In acceptance, you may be quiet and even somewhat withdrawn. At this stage, you become almost passive from time to time. You will find yourself eager to follow directions and ask for help. You won't be embarrassed. You will appear calm and inspire serenity and tranquility in others. You won't have "answers." Instead, you will be open to follow new directions. At this stage there is actually little to say or do. All you need is to sit back and enjoy the ride.

EXERCISE: ACCEPTING ACCEPTANCE

Check the feelings you have had within the past year.

I really don't have much confidence that this can be cured. _____

I think this will go on forever. _____

I'm sort of removed from all that. _____

I really don't seem affected any more by whether they like me or not. _____

If I don't keep my abstinence, all else feels miserable. _____

I see how much of my past emotion was generated by food. _____

I certainly won't waste my time in therapy if I'm still eating. _____

I see food has been my major tranquilizer and coping mechanism. _____

I wonder what my real life will be without bingeing. _____

I wonder what I'll do with excess time. _____

I feel somewhat withdrawn and quiet. _____

I don't have a clue whether I will really make it with this illness or not. _____

Family members are angry; I do not seem as jovial as I used to be. _____

I am feeling serene and quiet. _____

My feelings seem cut off and I am void. _____

I need to feel quiet. _____

Different things are becoming important and meaningful in my life. _____

What used to seem important now appears trivial. _____

I am not interested in anything but my recovery. _____

My abstinence is the most important thing in my life, without exception. _____

When you begin to accept the disease concept, the mind is open to new ideas, and you will show a childlike receptivity. You will come to know on a very deep level that *your own* efforts got you to exactly this place. You will find yourself willing to accept help from someone else. You'll know you can't do it alone. You'll ask for help. Men with broken legs can ask for crutches. With this disease, your prescription is "turn on to people." That is acceptance. You will become willing to live your life "one day at a time." You will give up previous fantasies. Realistic recovery is now fully underway.

In the beginning of acceptance, you may appear void of feelings and closed off. You must allow yourself this space. Codependents will need guidance and comfort to keep from rescuing.

You will not be interested in anything but recovery for a while. You will see that as the eating falls in line, all the other aspects of your life do, too. Your attitude must become "abstinence is the most important thing in life, *without exception.*"

Acceptance is not achieved once and for all. It is a process of surrender. It is not a destination. You'll see that you have to change relationships in order to survive. You do not necessarily go through these stages in a particular order, nor do you finish with one stage, never to return. It is a continuing and fluid process. Actually, the analogy to stages traveled in accepting death is not really far-fetched. In reality, you are laying to rest an old way of life and giving birth to a new personality. The process is often slow, but the timing is accurately paced for each one of us. You needn't worry about getting on with it or pushing too quickly. You have the rest of your life to travel these stages.

Often at this stage, other people become angry with you. They will see you are experiencing a significant change, and feel threatened that they are left out. Fortunately, you won't be attending to their feelings very much. They may be jealous that your recovery plan is working. As an E-D, many of the new ideas you learn about yourself are the very same things your codependent has been saying for years. They may wonder, "Why are you listening to *them* when you wouldn't listen to *me?*"

As a codependent you'll see your loved one listening and hearing, but moving away from you. As close as you are, you are least likely to be the helper. Each of you must work it out separately. You will each need a helper outside the family. You can get close again later. Let yourselves cry over the brief separation with the knowledge of a closeness beyond your imagination later on.

In the next chapter, you will see how both the E-D and codependent can turn to groups like Overeaters Anonymous and O-Anon for help. Once there is true acceptance of the need for help, you will see how to get it. This will help you extend the family system and develop some individuality so you can come back together healthier, closer, and stronger.

Chapter Six

Extend the Family System

To start a diet at this point would be another suicidal effort at control. Remember, your life experience has already demonstrated that diets don't do it. Instead, you must find a way to work with someone else to "relate to recover." Recovery will involve moving away from an obsessive relationship with food *or* your loved ones and toward nurturance from others outside your immediate system.

In this chapter you will find a way out of enmeshment and failed attempts at control, and into a more relaxed self-acceptance and ability to give and receive help from others. Your enmeshed family relationships will be traded for a more "distant" intimacy which will ultimately prove more healing.

MACHO MYTHS

Many of us live with the myth of total independence, i.e., "self-made man," "pulled up by your own bootstraps," "stiff upper lip," etc. Each of the braggardly proclamations can cost five to ten pounds. Instead of seeking mutual support, interdependence, and reliance on our friends, we eat! Sometimes we pay a therapist $100.00 an hour to listen. We really show the dependence we fear, but paying helps ease the shame and thus makes it more acceptable.

There is another way to gain effective support, nurturance, and understanding totally free of charge on a 24-hour-a-day basis, not just during business hours. You can extend your family system and get support outside the home. That support comes from Overeaters Anonymous for the E-D and O-Anon for the family and friends of E-Ds, the codependents. In some localities where O-Anon meetings may not be readily available, codependents may attend Al-Anon meetings which are for families and friends of alcoholics. The types of relationship patterns are similar enough. The E-D is addicted to solid sugar, while the alcoholic is addicted to liquid sugar. The meetings address not the substance, but the relationship.

Attend a meeting, humble yourself, and admit the need for help. Realize that you've already asked for this help hundreds of times before with doctor's visits, shots, pills, or fad diets. Now you are asking for another kind of help.

You are actually finding a way to rejoin the human race. You need to accept yourself and your plight as part of the human condition. You are not a weirdo or a freak. You have been trying to negotiate the difficult human dilemma of seeking nurturance without violation. You chose the safety of food, and now need to learn there is safety with people.

The people in Overeaters Anonymous are fallible human beings like yourself and therefore may, from time to time, "fail" you. Because you will be extending your neediness to a group rather than one or two individuals, you will be able to weather the disappointments.

"WE KNOW HOW HARD IT IS"

There is nothing easy about asking for help. Even some of the most motivated, open, willing people I've seen were scared to death to show their vulnerability. After all, you wouldn't have chosen an eating disorder if you were secure and open. This time you'll take a risk without your best friend. Just going to a meeting is a very risky proposition. It is both an admission that you can't fix it all alone, and a plea for help. What happens if they can't fix you right away? You want the quickie. What if they won't understand? The greatest fear is, "They wanna take my food away." You think you still need the old relationship with food.-

You may fear someone will actually take your "self" away. You sense that *you* have to change, not just your food. Don't worry, you won't give up more than you can surrender and you don't have to "throw away the baby with the bath water." This is a gradual shedding of the old way of life as you slowly learn new behaviors and attitudes. There is no hurry. You have the rest of your life to recover.

EMPATHY AND SYMPATHY

Just because O.A. members understand how hard it is does not mean they will do it for you. It means they can show you the way out and warn you of the pitfalls. The work is still yours to do. Your own family felt too responsible to let you sink or swim on your own. Whether enabling or punishing, they implied it was their job to fix you. At the O.A. meetings you will get support and guidance, but people there are committed to finding a way out; they seek solutions rather than reasons or excuses. Since the group comprises people who have struggled out of the depths of degradation, they know from first hand experience that it is difficult, but not impossible. In this new "family" system you will get support and encouragement and many necessary pats on the back, but no one will do your work for you. As Carl Jung said, "There is no birth of consciousness without pain." This is your chance to be reborn psychologically within the same physical lifetime. Overeaters Anonymous groups will become your powerful extended family. When you struggled to be born physically, your mother helped, but you struggled and pushed to move yourself out into this new life. Now you'll take on a new psychological birth. Group members will give you a lot of push and cheer you on, but the work is yours.

GETTING TO A MEETING

One advantage enjoyed by hospitalized patients is that we actually transport them to Overeaters Anonymous meetings. It would certainly be easier to just recommend they go, and leave it up to them. My experience has shown, however, that people will rarely follow that suggestion. They assure me they think it is a good idea and that they have every intention of going, but it is often months before they finally do. Don't let that be your situation. You are not hospitalized and there is no one hauling you to a meeting. You will have to push yourself to go. Don't sit at home reading this book and agreeing that it is a good idea. You won't know that until you go.

"Where do I go?" The easiest way to find your first meeting is by calling information and asking for Overeaters Anonymous. From that call you can also find out about O-Anon for codependents. If you have trouble, place a long distance call to the World Headquarters of O.A. in Torrance, California at 213-320-7941. They maintain an updated directory for the entire world and can give you a local meeting place as well as names and telephone numbers of people to call in your community. You may call these people to get directions to your local meeting and even transportation should you need it. The people who have their phone numbers listed are offering themselves to help newcomers, and will gladly help get you to your first meeting. You can call the local O.A. office and ask them to send you a directory of local meetings. The directory will give addresses of meetings, times, and contact persons with phone numbers. LET'S GO!!!

After the preliminary introductions are out of the way, Marva says, "Last night I saw how much my mom uses me for a garbage can. She dumps on me all the stuff she really needs to be saying to my dad. She's been doing it since I was sixteen, telling me about her affairs and attractions to other men and stuff because Dad is supposedly so 'closed up.' I wish she'd tell *him* that instead of me. I'm the one who gets all her venom and deceits but with Dad she pretends and makes nice! She complains about their relationship, but she sure seems to like it this way. I can release the tension I pick up from her by bingeing my brains out and then vomiting! I'm tired. I've got to tell her we can't be confidantes anymore and I can't listen to her stuff. It's not my job! Let her deal with her husband or go see her own therapist. I've got my own life to live!"

No one responds; there is no "cross talk" at the O.A. meeting. Members use the group as a forum to "go public" with their private thoughts and feelings. They realize their eating disorders are diseases of isolation; that by sharing their innermost selves they can stop turning to food for solace. No one is asking for advice, just a "witness." They need each other to witness their own personal growth journey. The presence of others is comforting. During "sharing," each person gets to hear a personal echo. They hear themselves as they share with others.

At meetings, people talk about things they would not mention elsewhere. Each has made a commitment to try to stop eating compulsively. Not eating produces a need to let out feelings that bubble up.

Annette speaks next: "It's really hard to tell my husband I'm bored. He lets me make all our party and social plans. I carry on all the discussions with our kids and manage our entire lives. That was great when I was eating compulsively. It was my perfect excuse for overeating. After all, I'd say, I have to care for all these other people. I want my reward. My reward was food. Now that food is out of my picture, I want more from those I love. I'm finding out they're not there for me. The only place I feel nurtured is when I come to these meetings."

Arthur, a very obese young man, pipes up angrily from the back of the room. "My mom is a perfect earth mother and I love her. I wouldn't want her coming to a meeting! She'd get her head filled with all these ideas about taking care of yourself. As it is now, she pays my bills when I get in a jam, she gets my dirty socks out from under the bed and makes sure they're washed and matched. She likes it this way and so do I. I'm just here to lose a little weight. Why change a perfectly workable family situation? What's the difference who manages whose life?"

Arthur doesn't expect an answer. He knows it's okay to blow off some steam and express himself. There are no judgments. Feelings are neither "right" nor "wrong." They just *are*. By hearing himself speak, Arthur is free to dig in his position, change his mind, or simply do nothing. This is the ideal family environment. Members get heard but not lectured.

The members do care about what happens to each other. They have a common illness and know how hard it is to open up and also how crucial it is for survival. It would be terrible to criticize or judge each other for speaking openly. Each is there to witness the other. If they want feedback or further discussion, they can ask specific people after the meeting or confide in their sponsor, the person they've chosen to be their guide through the recovery process. They've learned to "relate to recover."

Before getting to O.A., they had all tried changing their food instead of their lives. Their best efforts walked them through the doors of their first meeting. They had dieted their way up to 200 or 400 pounds. Some are thin or normal. They eat and then vomit, or abuse laxatives. By the time they got to that first meeting, most found they ate for any reason. Whether in celebration or mourning, there is always good reason to eat. They now come to these meetings for an experience that often can't be explained. That's okay, what they get keeps them from food. Though they can't explain what they get, they know it works and satisfaction with self lasts while the compulsion to eat drifts away. Their slogan is, "If it works, don't fix it."

What is the healing process and what can you as a reader gain from attending these meetings? The meetings offer a forum for self-expression and an opportunity to open up and be seen. The avoidance of that visibility is what hiding in food is all about. Instead, meetings bring you out. Meetings work as a form of reparenting. Children need a witness. Little Johnny plays on the sliding board and shouts, "Look Daddy, watch me go!" Daddy doesn't know what to do or say; he responds as his father did, "That's a great slide." This scenario certainly meets all the guidelines for effective parenting. We see Dad providing positive support and encouragement as well as praise. However, we miss one crucial point: WHO ASKED HIM? No one asked for his praise, encouragement, or evaluation. Johnny only asked for a witness. "Watch me Daddy." That's all. Unfortunately, most of us don't know how to be good watchers or listeners. We feel we have to offer something and give in order to feel adequate and valuable. Who asked? At Overeaters Anonymous meetings, members get *witnessed*. That's the healing process. That's the new relating. The meeting provides you the audience you need in order to come out. Happy Birthday!

CONDUCT OF A MEETING

These meetings will be your place for YOU. You will eventually come to see this group of people as an extended family. Therefore, go to a meeting with an attitude of making it your place. Here, as nowhere else, will be a place you can be totally yourself. Whatever you say or do will be okay. Above all, don't try to make an impression or influence others. This is your place to be cared for and nurtured. Save your impressive stuff for the rest of the world. Let your little self emerge here. I suggest you attend initially as an observer/listener. Save your questions until you have attended at least three meetings. Try to go at first just to listen and learn.

Most meetings run for an hour or two, depending on the format and local preferences. There is usually a written procedure for conduct of the meeting. This provides structure for the leader for that day. Most groups do not have established regular leaders, but shift this role to new people each week.

There are few DOs and DON'Ts about behavior at meetings. It is intended as a place for you to be spontaneous and be yourself. There is only one cardinal rule suggested at most meetings. That is: "NO CROSS TALK." Members are encouraged to talk about *themselves* and *their own* experiences, but offer no advice to others about what they should or shouldn't do. In other words, you are safe to express your own feelings without others telling you what to do. Those who talk are talking to hear their own echo. The purpose of self-expression is self-expression. Often, by hearing what comes out of your mouth, you gain an understanding of how you feel. Then you'll instinctively know the right actions for you.

You may drop in late and leave early. You can do whatever works and fits your life. There will be no demands made on you by O.A. The best advice is "take what you can use, and leave the rest." Don't get attached to many questions. Let them all pass for now.

TYPES OF MEETINGS

Meetings are different in different parts of the country. They are composed of different types of people with varying attitudes. You will find the same cross sections of people there that you find anywhere. A specific meeting can change from week to week. Therefore, I recommend you try one meeting at least three times. See the variations. Inspect, don't reject. After all, haven't you given food a second chance? Remember when something tasted slightly moldy? Didn't you take another taste just to make sure? Only then did you reluctantly toss it out. Give the same second chance to this recovery program which can save your life. Codependents have given controlling and destructive behavior patterns more than a second or third chance. You doggedly held onto old behaviors insisting that "just one more time" would work. Try to develop the same type of faith in attending meetings. It's a way to help you detach from the E-D and get help for yourself. It's a way to come back home.

Allowing for all the possible differences, here is a brief outline of the types of meetings you can expect.

Speaker Meeting. Speakers vary from meeting to meeting. At a speaker meeting, one member presents an hour-long talk about how they've been helped. These are not professional speakers, simply fellow members of the group. They are advised to talk about what their lives had been like, how they found a way out, and what their lives are like now. Some meetings allow for question and answer time, but usually the speaker stops and then others can speak for themselves.

Pitch Meeting. Anyone in the group can volunteer to speak. No one has to speak. Each speaker talks for three to five minutes. They may talk about anything; usually topics are current activities or something they are learning about themselves or others. There is no cross-talk or commenting.

Discussion Meeting. Members sit in a circle and discuss a specific topic decided by the group or the leader. Even if a topic is named, members can still talk about anything they like. The format is relaxed and open and each member can talk as many times as time allows.

Book Study. A number of books recommended by the O.A. fellowship are read at specific meetings. Sometimes these are books from Alcoholics Anonymous. Members are asked to read a paragraph and then discuss how it applies to them. Each person's opinion is her or his own interpretation. Sometimes all members at the meeting can discuss how the particular paragraph applies to them.

Writing Meeting. The group agrees to a specific topic, and then members write about it. Later, some may read their written work to the group. At some meetings there is response from other group members, and at some there is reading with no comments invited.

Newcomer's Meeting. In many cities, especially large metropolitan centers, special meetings are organized for beginners, where specifics of the program are explained. A member introduces basic concepts about the treatment plan and is then available to answer questions and offer suggestions to the newcomer. Remember, O.A. is not run by professionals in the eating disorders field, but by fellow recovering members who can advise about what worked *for them*. Notice this book does not provide elaborate detail or explanation about the treatment plan of O.A.. It is instead suggested that you *go* to the meetings and then use exercises in this book as an adjunct. You will learn all you need to know as you attend.

Directories. When you call a local group center in your locality, request a directory of local meetings be sent to you. You can also pick up a directory at your first meeting. These will list the types of meetings offered as well as the name and phone number of a contact person should you like more information before attending. GO AHEAD AND MAKE THAT CALL. You have nothing to lose but your obsession with food. If you don't like the meetings they'll refund your misery.

THE NEW FAMILY SYSTEM

Whatever type of meeting you choose, you will come to see the people there as a new family for you. Many have proclaimed after a meeting, "I've come *home* at last! No one ever understood me like these people. I can talk about anything I like, and someone else feels that way, too." "Whatever I say, I am accepted and feel worthwhile." "I love how no one tells me what to do." "I'm not alone as a freak anymore!"

The most important healing ingredient of the O.A. program is the meeting. This is what cures the loneliness and isolation. E-Ds and codependents are needy people with fluid and changing ego boundaries. Each needs support and encouragement. Depending on just one other person to fill those needs is insufficient. You need the group. You need to spread around those needs. In that way, you learn to weather rejection without food. If one person is busy, or can't be there for you right that minute, there is always someone else in the group. You won't have to be alone. Loneliness leads back to food. Including others leads out of addiction. You will find it becomes more fun to be with people than with food. The choice will be very clear and much less painful. As people get closer, food will become boring. I can reassure you, we're really gonna mess up your relationship with food. You just can't eat in the same old way anymore. Sorry.

SCIENCE CATCHES UP

Professional research in the treatment of eating disorders is rapidly catching up with methods practiced in Overeaters Anonymous for the past twenty-four years. In October of 1983, research projects reported at the Fourth International Obesity Congress in New York City showed that two crucial elements of the O.A. program are also proving most effective in professional treatment. They include treating people in groups rather than individually, and peer counseling, that is, one fellow sufferer helping another. Every research project mentioned showed that people did much better in a group than individually. Even when the "treatment" was dispensing a placebo pill, those who took the pill in a group setting had more success than those who took the pill alone. Also, a study at Vanderbilt University showed that when one group of patients, more advanced, was asked to work as the counselors for the second group, dropout rates were practically eliminated and weight loss results were 85 percent higher! As medical science continues to catch up with programs like O.A., we will see more research explaining why these methods work. For now, we can just take it on faith that if it has worked for so many others, it can work for you.

REPARENTING

E-Ds and codependents came by their behaviors and feelings quite honestly. You did the best you could with what you knew then and what you had to work with. What was missing was a chance to remain a child. You grew up too quickly, so as to parent your own parent. Now it's time for you to collect on the parenting. You need parents who understand and respect you and expect nothing from you. Both E-Ds and codependents need a place to become children again. In your new O.A. or O-Anon family, no one really expects anything of you. It's up to you to give what you want. You don't owe anyone anything. Actually, for quite a while, the only expectation is that you be the receiver—the BABY. Newcomers in O.A. are referred to as "babies." Members actually celebrate "birthdays" as the day they entered O.A. and, essentially, were born into a new way of life. You are expected to be like a newborn babe. Don't push yourself to learn, grow, or achieve. Instead, relax into your recovery. You don't have to worry about learning it all right away. You have the rest of your life to recover.

Your new parent figure in O.A. will be someone you call a "sponsor." The sponsor is another member who you, as a newcomer, pick for yourself. You believe you can learn from them. You must make the first move and ask someone to be your sponsor. No one will push themselves on you; they don't want to violate you in any way. They will wait until you ask for help. Of course, you know how hard *that* is, and so do they. Look and listen at the meetings and try to find someone who you think you can talk with, someone who could offer you guidance. Members recommend, "Find someone who has what you want." If you admire what they've done with their lives, ask them for guidance so you can do the same.

Different things attract different people. Some want only to talk with someone who has been as fat as they have. One patient told me, "I don't want to bother with anyone who hasn't lost at least a hundred pounds." Others discriminate by looking for the correct eating pattern that matched theirs, such as other vomiters, or week-end bingers.

Your reasons for choosing a sponsor aren't as important as just choosing someone so you can get started on the journey. *That* is the healing ingredient. When you choose a sponsor you are investing in your recovery. It's a step toward asking for help. That's the hard part. You may change sponsors when you like and you may end up having many sponsors throughout your recovery. People change and grow and move in different directions. The Hindus say, "When the student is ready, the teacher appears." Don't worry about picking the sponsor. You will choose exactly who you need and what you are ready for right now.

MUTUAL TRUST AND INTERDEPENDENCE

The sponsor/baby relationship is the crucial healing ingredient in recovery. Previously a "terminally unique" case which aborted treatment, you come to this relationship both asking for help and investing yourself in the recovery process. It is clear no one else will fix you or even expects you to be fixed. With the sponsor, you will not have the excessively enmeshed relationship you had in your own family. You were all too close to help. In this new relationship there will be enough distance to keep it safe, but a new closeness as you share a common undertaking. You will become "survivors" together and have reminiscences similar to GIs who shared the trenches of war. No one else will understand the rigors of hell you suffer as you transfer dependency on food to a new relationship with other people. Nowhere will you get more for giving less.

Nadia had a lifelong dream which richly illustrates the E-D's longing for nurturance. Her dream never became a reality, so she ate instead. This same dream came to her at least eight times a year and upon awakening, she cried. In this dream, Nadia was a one-celled organism, an amoeba. This single-celled amoeba was three feet in diameter, an undulating, fluid body mass. Tiny hairlike growths radiated from the outer circumference. The interior fluid was a rich transparent green like gooey hairset lotion. This gigantic cell slithered quickly, adjusting its form as it went. This was Nadia. She recounted the recurring dream as if *she* was the amoeba:

> *I feel particularly heavy and slow. I am grotesque. When I move, I blob along from side to side feeling listless and heavy. I feel like wherever the weight of my "goo" pulls me, the rest follows. I blob and slither slowly into a room full of people. I hear faint murmurs of their reactions as they move out of my way. They jump back aghast with "eeeeeeeeooooooooo" and "yech" and "ick, creepy" but I keep on coming. I feel sorry for all of them because they have to look at me and I know I am revolting. I suck myself up off the floor into one of the chairs. I work hard to get up the chair leg and then feel depleted. I melt into the chair. Parts of me hang over the sides of the folding chair. I heave a giant sigh and settle myself to rest. The people in the room eventually stop staring at me and continue with their own business. Quite unexpectedly, a young woman moves out of the blur of strange faces and figures and comes over to sit in the chair beside me. I am still and scared. I stop breathing. No longer undulating in and out, I remain perfectly still in shock. I want to disappear, but know I attract more attention trying to move. I rest and keep still and pray no one will look. The next thing I know, she reaches over and starts petting me on my hairy back. With soft determined strokes, she continues, not even noticing how slimy I am. I'm shocked! She continues long after she should be repulsed. I start to relax, figuring she really doesn't notice what she's touching. Soon I relax fully into the experience and even feel like cooing I'm so blissful. No one has ever petted me like that. She seems to be touching me just because*

she likes me. How weird, I thought. What does she get out of this? Shouldn't I be doing something in return? What's the payback? She just keeps on petting. I coo. Then I wake up.

That same kind of experience is what many report from their first O.A. meeting. They find that same kind of acceptance, nurturance, and support. What's odd is, nothing's *expected.* You are accepted for just coming in the door. After that, "just have a seat and relax." Nadia's dream represents her lifelong search for unconditional love. Even at her most repulsive, she longs for acceptance without having to earn it. "Love me, love my fat." In O.A., the E-D has a chance to be bathed in acceptance regardless of production.

The sponsor's message is, "it is hard enough to refrain from eating compulsively. You really don't have to put on any airs or act any roles here. O.A. is where you can come home to fall apart. Have a seat and relax. You *can* be passive here."

What happens between you and your sponsor is as varied as the members of O.A. You will have to trust that the directions you are given are meant with love and your best interests at heart. The sponsor will tell you, "If you want what I have, you must do what I do." The sponsor will recommend certain things that have worked for her or him. These are suggestions, not orders. Feel free to argue with your sponsor. That is the way to have a healthy relationship. You must share your resistance. Blindly following won't work, as you will soon slip away when you have a disagreement. Totally rejecting all the sponsor's suggestions is also a waste of time. You will find the middle ground of trusting someone else as well as trusting yourself.

Don't let your criticisms go underground and don't just smile and tell everyone how wonderful you think the meetings are. I have seen many proclaiming the value of O.A. meetings and their ultimate joy in attending. Then they just stop going. What happened? They didn't know how to express their criticisms. You are bound to have criticisms. After all, you are facing the reality of turning around your entire life and doing things in a whole new way. All your relationships in the world will change. You are bound to balk. Let's balk out loud.

Trust your reactions. They indicate where you are right now. Listed below are some of the thoughts and feelings of others. Notice the broad range of responses and all the variations and contradictions.

Compare these with your own. You may uncover a pattern as your own reactions change dramatically from the first to the fourth meeting. That is why you will hear, at the end of each meeting, "KEEP COMING BACK."

Most suffer an approach/avoidance reaction to their first meetings. You want what they have, but are also scared to death to reach out. In this way, you will appreciate having found a place to feel accepted and understood, and, at the same time, try to pick it apart and find fault. This is a natural reaction to the threat of change. Let yourself flow with that. Here are some comments from patients after returning from their first meetings.

WHAT DID YOU LEARN AT THE MEETING?

"One day at a time."
Too many rules for me.
I feel hostile.
I feel like I can open up to these people.
Others have it worse than I do.
I am not alone.
I have feelings like the speaker.
I really am out of control.
I see how hard it is.
It's not about food, but you can't forget food.
I see the illness is about relating in the world.
These people are a snotty bunch.
I think they're phony. I don't like all the hugging.
I'm so shy.
I learned it's a disease and I'm powerless.
Don't eat, no matter what. This too shall pass.
I feel very sorry for myself.
I don't like the seriousness of all this.
I feel uneasy. I've never had it as bad as they do.
I hate myself for being here.
I applaud myself for sticking out the meeting.
I feel like all these people are closing in on me.
I'm angry. I want to kick everyone.
I don't feel like working this hard on this stuff.
I thought one of the guys was cute.
People talk real honestly here.

Even though they've come to a meeting, some people are still jerks.
I was scared to talk, but afterwards felt high.
I felt like an observer rather than a member.
I see I, too, have something to give, not just take.
Recovery *is* possible.
I know I weighed over 200 pounds. I have the pictures, but when
    I get around other E-Ds I want to deny it.
I'm afraid.
I feel the strength of the others in recovery.
I can see how I try to reject the help.
I chose a new sponsor today and I feel excited.
I entered the meeting feeling resentful and now I leave feeling peaceful
    and calm.
I see how much I'd rather help others than care for myself.
I get scared to talk in front of the men.
I hate how they see themselves as such givers!
I need to learn to mind my own business.
This is treatment. Nothing is more important.
I thought about tomorrow's meals throughout the whole meeting.
I see how it's a family disease.
I liked the small group. It forced me to come out of myself.
We don't know each other, but I can tell they understand.
I can't stand the smoke.
I see how being married doesn't "fix" you either.
I like the jokes.
I can see I don't have to play at being a nice person.
I see whether I eat or not, the problem will still be there.
I don't like all those slogans and catch-phrases.
A man told me "you look radiant" and it scared me to death!
I've got to keep my eyes off him and on myself.

CAPITALIZE THE CRITIC

Most critical comments about the meetings fall into three major
areas, the WOUNDED HEALERS, DISORGANIZATION, AND
RELIGIOUSNESS. Let's take a look at these major blocks to the
program.
    Wounded Healers. There is often concern that the people at
the meetings are "just as sick" as those seeking help. That's right.

That's exactly why the program is so effective. People identify their own strengths and weaknesses by observing others with similar afflictions. This, of course, is the prevalent concept in group psychotherapy; that we learn from watching others grow. Often another sufferer can notice an addict's denial system and self-delusion more clearly than the addict. A therapist friend of mine was treating an overeater who she asked each week, "How's your food?" The client dutifully reported with a smile, "Fine." This went on for months but the patient put on 60 pounds! Another addict is often much more attuned to the delusion of the denial system. They know to ask for more specifics and closer scrutiny of the daily food plan. They help you remove those personal blinders we all have when we choose not to see. This may sound inviting, but also terrifying.

Along this line, critical newcomers complain O.A. members are "too sick" to help them. Their complaint is that "I'm not that bad. I've never gotten that fat or been that obsessed, or vomited that often. Those people are really sickos. Not for me."

This refrain often comes from a person who has a minimal acquaintance with the obsession and is in the early stages. They don't want to believe that, to recover, they will have to get honest and show parts of themselves they don't like. This is particularly true for the bingers who vomit. They work at all costs to look good. They are, therefore, very judgmental of people who show weakness. To avoid showing themselves, they develop a case of what is called the *yets*. "I haven't done that *yet*. I'm not that bad *yet*. That hasn't happened to me *yet*." The yets help them stay critical of others. They will have to go through a lot more pain before they can accept help. If you notice yourself veering toward the yets, try to ask yourself why you should have to go that far down the road before you are ready to turn around? Why not get help now, instead of suffering more? Try to think of those who have suffered before you as "scouts" warning you of the dangers ahead. Maybe you can head some of your suffering off at the pass if you become willing to participate earlier. The yets are just a delaying action. Why not grab on now?

Disorganization. Rejections of O.A. because of structure problems include both ends of the spectrum. Either the group is "too controlling, excessively rigid and demanding, with no flexibility or humanity," or else it's "too haphazard, they don't start on time, everyone does their own thing with no definite structure or direction."

It's all true. So what? As an E-D or codependent, you have a lot of conflict over control, aggression, and passivity. You are keenly adept at discovering loopholes in the control and organization of groups. After all, the people in O.A. have difficulty being disciplined and keeping commitments to themselves, so they would just naturally take these same traits into their group meetings. That, however, is not cause to leave the meeting. Instead, it is a good training ground for you to experience living with "too much" or "too little" organization. Some complain they want to be ordered what to do. Others complain that the group is "too bossy." In O.A. you will learn to follow directions from fallible human beings. The issue for the newcomer is, can you give up control and follow directions? Can you trust that this must be what you need right now? "When the student is ready, the teacher appears."

Religiousness. In my seventeen years of treating addictive personalities, one criticism I've heard of meetings stands out above all others. Whether a narcotic addict, an overeater, or a professional in the field, the readily available criticism is, "There's too much God talk. I'm not religious." In fact, O.A. is a spiritual program, not religious. Consider the possibility that you are actually very religious. You have been worshipping an external substance which you believed could cure your ills and solve your problems. Food was God. In recovery you will look for something less destructive to believe in. You don't need to adopt a God concept. You may instead look and listen for your own "still, small voice within." That is your own personal God you've been ignoring. When you keep yourself sedated and self-loathing with food, you can't pay attention to the special messages from within. That is why I say we are as fat as we are dishonest. The degree to which we have refused to follow directions from our own personal message center is the degree to which we have to worship food. By attending these meetings, you will give up the obsession with food and find a way to live more closely attuned to your own internal voice. Call it God or call it chopped liver. Whether a rose or a thorn by name, it works.

COMMITMENT

There are a number of suggested and recommended food plans in O.A. and I don't believe any one to be better than another. What matters is the commitment you make regarding eating behavior. The crucial ingredient is the commitment. The agenda is to change relationships, and a changed food plan will follow. This works when the newcomer makes a morning decision about what will be eaten that day and writes it down. The food plan can be as varied as the weather, events of the day, or personal preferences. Each day is taken anew, one day at a time. The newcomer "baby" then calls the sponsor with the plan. Sponsors are not trained nutritionists, but rather fellow sufferers who have been successful. They may or may not advise or comment. Their major role is to serve as a witness to your commitment to yourself. They are neither your judge nor your disciplinarian; they are your confidantes who will listen as you promise yourself something. You may easily break a promise to yourself, but hesitate to break promises to others. With this commitment, you are including someone else in your thought process, and your obsession with food. Of all the recommendations to newcomers, the idea of sharing the food commitment with someone else is often an insurmountable stumbling block. Most people absolutely hate this idea of calling in food. Protests range from seeing it as childish, punitive, a waste of time, an imposition on someone else, to stupid and unnecessary, and generally inconvenient. It is difficult because it involves imposing some control and discipline on your relationship with food. It is an intrusion to bring someone else into that most intimate and private relationship. "How dare they look at my plate! I'm not a child." But you are a child where food is concerned. Remember, your sponsor will be a new parent figure, not punitive, just guiding.

THE DAY AFTER

Some people who attend their first meeting fall madly in love with Overeaters Anonymous and decide food is no longer an issue in their lives. They get joy from being with other E-Ds, they feel miraculously cured and finished with obsessions. They have arrived! That, however, is not what really happens. In the therapy field we call this a "flight into health." The person has become frightened by the amount of work in store and say "everything's wonderful, my problems are over." What they are really saying is, "thanks a lot Doc. It's been great. See 'ya later," and "PHEW, got outta that one." They are again believing in the "quickie." Members of O.A.

call this the honeymoon period. You want to believe you've found the way. Actually, you have, but there's still work to do.

More usual than the flight into health is the immediate rejection of O.A. You may find very good reasons why this is not the place for you. Rejecting the meetings often happens because, as George Bernard Shaw quipped many years ago, "I don't want to be a member of any club that would have *me* as a member." You may decide the entrance requirements are too liberal. You want a more exclusive club. Perhaps one that is more familiar to you. Both E-Ds and codependents tend to use the same types of excuses for rejecting meetings. Initially proclaiming it's a great idea, you can then decide it just doesn't seem right for you. No matter what the excuse, you actually fear being vulnerable and seeking help from other fallible human beings. You will try at all costs to protect yourself from being human and vulnerable.

THREATS TO THE OLD WITH PROMISE OF NEW

In any system there is a strong pull to keep the status quo. Stability is easier than change, even if change promises something better. That is true for obese bodies. They slow down their metabolism to stay fat even when the brain decides to go on a diet. The same commitment to the status quo holds for the family system. Even if the old ways served to keep the E-D obsessed with food and the codependent obsessed with the E-D, there will be a strong tendency to maintain the old ways instead of trying something new. Many have the idea that "our family problems are our own and we'll solve them ourselves." Remember, your best efforts got you where you are right now. You must realize that trying a new way will be a threat to the past, an admission that the old way didn't work. You will start the detachment process, and it is threatening because it is new.

SUPPORT FOR SANITY

By continuing to attend these meetings, both E-Ds and codependents will learn to detach from one another and help themselves. You will each have your own sponsor for support and guidance, and will be willing to let those you love take care of themselves.

You will find yourself feeling more deserving and less guilty. You will realize that by keeping your eyes on yourself and your own plate, your whole family will develop separateness, so later you will be able to move back together stronger and more assertively.

RESISTANCE CHECKLIST

Check those you have often thought or said.

I can do it myself. _____
I am infallible. _____
I don't relate to those people. _____
They are too thin. _____
I don't want to be too thin. _____
They are depressing. _____
Those people are much "sicker" than I am. _____
They use foul language there. _____
They are too religious. _____
They are crazy. _____
I'm not that bad yet. _____
I don't like the food plan. _____
They have no food plan. _____
It's too vague and unstructured. _____
I don't like people telling me what to do. _____
There are no prizes. _____
I live too far to travel to those meetings. _____
Meetings are boring. _____
I can't telephone people. _____
Those people are too demanding. _____
I want more discussion as a group—cross-talk. _____
These meetings take time away from myself. _____
I went once and that's enough. _____
It's too simplistic. _____
I've already dealt with all those issues. _____
The meetings cause problems at home. _____
My spouse objects. _____
I don't need to hear other people's problems. _____
Boring. _____
Too scary to look at these problems.

The people are more sloppy, dumb, smart, loud, quiet (etc.)
   than I am.   _____
There are not enough direct solutions.   _____
Too many side discussions.   _____
They are having too much fun! Get serious!   _____
I really don't want to believe there is hope.   _____
They want to take my food away.   _____
The times are inconvenient.   _____
They don't give enough specifics on what to do.   _____

Chapter Seven

No to Food Is Yes to Life

In giving up the security of food and the enmeshment of smothering relationships, you are moving to a new flexibility and excitement about life and yourself. By attending meetings and sharing, you will begin to discover the self you drowned with food. Codependents will grow to respect themselves whether they are fixing someone or not. Your relationships will become more honest. You have to relate honestly or return to the food obsession.

THE BODY DOESN'T LIE

When you are neither bingeing nor starving compulsively, your body will be a perfect indicator of your own proper direction and course of action. Self-doubt will evaporate as you begin to listen for internal cues to let you know what is right. Your body will not lie. You will find an ability to gauge situations intuitively. Many have found this has profound effects on all relationships, especially intimate ones. How many have had sexual relations just because they seemed to have started something and weren't able to admit that "the mind is willing, but the body is not." Men have a clearer indicator of this deceit, as their bodies just won't operate when it's not ready. Women, on the other hand, have developed a keener ability to mask their ambivalence. For example, let's say that Prince Charming has just taken you to dinner at a fine, romantic place where you've always wanted to go. He's terrific. You just feel all close, warm, affectionate, and "ready." You're at home and alone and he picks up your signal and he's ready, too. As the clothes fly, the bed turns down, and you continue to embrace, your mind wanders innocently to a preoccupation with difficulties you had at work. Do you stop? Do you pause and whisper, "Dear, my mind just wandered and I started thinking about other things. Can we wait a few minutes?" How many are that honest with their sexuality?

More often, partners decide to follow through in order to "protect" the other's feelings. Whose feelings have been protected? Do you really believe your partner doesn't know you left the room? Maybe these things are never discussed, but in truth, the body knows when it's abandoned. It might be more loving to tell your partner you've left for a while. That can let you come back in honesty. It's not a personal affront. It's not malicious or insensitive. It's just honest, human, and the truth. Who could ask for more? If your organism signals to you that you aren't ready, then you aren't ready. There is no humane explanation for why people dishonestly pretend they're hot when they're not. There is really no logical reason to be dishonest in bed, except if we are concerned about weak egos and fragile self-concepts. In your new recovery programs, both you and your partner should be learning that you are much more than your image, and you both deserve the chance to be real. When you are saying no to the food obsession, you need to learn to say no to other things that are harmful to you, as well.

In this chapter, you will experience coming home again to your *self*. You will learn techniques to be more grounded and secure so you won't need the weight. Without this grounding, you'll get too scared. You'll return to excess food, and lost poundage will quickly reappear. Now is the time to say no to food and yes to your own life.

Tiffany was a budding Hollywood starlet, making every casting call and audition. She was also anorexic and a periodic vomiter. From time to time she landed a walk-on part or a brief appearance on the "soaps." Her career was just getting off the ground, but her vomiting was growing more excessive. She had even been talked into a few producer's beds. Tiffany accepted many of the dehumanizing aspects of her chosen career and began to use herself as a commodity.

She starved herself painfully for weeks at a time and then resorted to weekend "pigouts." She also vomited after every sexual foray with men she didn't like. "As an actor, I use *myself* as my instrument," she rationalized. "Everyone knows a great part of an actor's life is spent in 'seeking work' rather than working. This is just one of the methods I use for job hunting. And it works!" Tiffany had effectively rationalized behavior which was harmful to her.

Her body could not carry out the lie. The more she jumped in and out of Hollywood beds, the more she vomited in rage at what she "had to do" in order to work. When she asked for help with the vomiting, she found her sexual life had to change in order to change her relationship with food.

She had to learn how to say no. She also said no to the part of herself that told her she couldn't make it without violation and humiliation. She could no longer chide herself. Ultimately, for each person in recovery, the issue is the need to reevaluate choices in how to live. It's not just the eating pattern that has to change. Tiffany's decision came on a soap opera set during lunch. Alan was the star of the show and the latest heartthrob to millions of women. Everyone knew that he and his wife, Vanessa, had an "understanding" about his need to sleep around, both to further his career and so he wouldn't feel "cramped" or "tied down." He was a womanizer, but no matter where he wandered, his heart belonged to Vanessa; he'd never take anyone else seriously. Tiffany saw Alan as the perfect vehicle for furthering her career. She mapped out a plan that traded a closeness with Alan for a few more appearances on this particular soap. Everyone on the set, including writers, listened to what Alan wanted; he was the show's main attraction.

Tiffany set out to entice Alan to serve her interests. For two weeks, she slyly played just hard enough to get to make him very interested. She acted both coy and indifferent—he liked challenges. While in the midst of this seductive game, however, Tiffany began an abstinent food plan and a commitment to herself and her sponsor that she would not vomit. After only three days of abstaining from vomiting, Tiffany found herself becoming edgy, scared, and terribly angry. Her irritation came out at salesgirls who wouldn't answer her queries "intelligently," or waitresses who didn't move quickly enough for her. In the midst of this irritable stage, Alan sat down at her table. "I've been noticing you," he said, "and I can tell you've been noticing me."

"Of course I've noticed you. You're the star of the show."

"Well, I can also star in a number of other performances."

"So I've heard."

"How'd you like to give me an audition? No strings attached. I really like seeing you around here."

This was just the proposition Tiffany had been working toward. It clearly offered promise of furthering her career. However, without either the excess food to bolster her bravado, or the outlet of vomiting to relieve her self-disgust and rage, Tiffany's answer had to come out differently.

"No thanks, I want to play a starring role in my own life." The words flowed out of her from somewhere deep within. "Your wife has top billing in your play, and I want the same billing in my own life." With that first refusal, Tiffany set out on a new career path and a new feeling about herself. The elation she felt at taking the risk of saying no to Alan buoyed her up for days. Before this, the only highs she felt were the euphoric feelings of power she had after starving. Now she felt strong and confident and very excited about the riskiness of it all. He might be offended and want her off the set. She might never work again! Who knew? All Tiffany knew was that she had to say no to preserve her abstinence. She couldn't handle those quick trysts without bingeing and vomiting. Her behavior was determined by her abstinence.

Saying no to Alan did not hurt Tiffany's career. The writers and director saw her value to the show, and she was written in for two more months. They were impressed with the strength of character she brought to her part. Now that she was no longer hiding her vomiting, Tiffany was able to freely show all of herself. She had no secrets and nothing to hide. Today she's a star and she came by it honestly and abstinently.

Tiffany is one of thousands who have said no to some parts of their old lives in order to say yes to abstinence and recovery. This chapter will teach you how to say no and feel okay about it. You will learn to play a starring role in your own life with a healthier cast of supporting characters. Most of us are initially scared of starring in our own lives, let alone actually directing them. Giving up the power to say "no" and the ability to direct your own life is what keeps you bingeing and self-destructing—because it's a lie. Every time we say yes when we need to say no, we are lying. The only way to live a lie is to eat. A good way to avoid sitting down to an excessive meal is learning to stand up for *yourself.*

You have spent a large part of this book taking stock of your situation and how you got here. You have looked at your personality and traced the stages you and your loved ones go through to achieve lasting recovery. Now it is time to practice new ways to handle old situations which will help you feel comfortable and stay abstinent. You'll say no to food and yes to life.

E-Ds and codependents each swing back and forth on the pendulum between passivity and aggressiveness. Neither has achieved the moderation of assertiveness. Many people without an eating disorder can live their whole lives without ever changing these parts of themselves. They don't have to change their roles in life. They never have to practice assertiveness. E-Ds and codependents can't afford the luxury. How you behaved previously has kept you eating. Change or eat, these are the choices.

FAT LADIES ARE GIANT "THANK YOU" CARDS

You have to be. You are busy overcompensating for your grotesqueness. You feel morally inferior and legally guilty. You are slavishly grateful for any crumbs of human kindness and actually encourage others to punish rather than reward you. Therefore, if anyone treats you well, you need to make it up to them by paying back a thousandfold.

When you give up eating compulsively you will find that much of this ingratiating behavior has to stop. You don't need to impress anyone because you aren't feeling guilty. You know you are doing the best you can about your illness, one day at a time. With nothing to hide and nowhere to run, you start feeling firm about what you can and can't do. In order to manage staying abstinent, you may have to slow down many of the tasks you previously performed so speedily and perfectly for others. Other achievements will recede as abstinence becomes of primary importance. This is bound to have effects on all your near and distant relationships.

As codependents you have adjusted well to the E-D as a guilty, self-loathing person. You will now have to change old behaviors. As codependents, you are sometimes ingratiating when you really feel angry. Together, one E-D and one codependent make up one whole, nurtured, responsible person. In recovery you each reclaim the missing part of yourself.

WHO'S ON CENTER?

Passivity and aggressiveness are intimately allied with eating disorders. Remember, the body doesn't lie. It is no accident that E-Ds have bodies that change shape almost as often as the weather. Your body is showing confusion at not knowing how to stand in the world. It undulates like a giant mushroom cloud pushing out to occupy more space and power and then rapidly shrinking again. Because you have not learned how to represent yourself adequately to others, you feel that amassing or diminishing flesh will create the effects you seek. Unfortunately, the body rarely catches up with how you truly feel about yourself. Saying no gives the body a leading edge on reality.

PASSIVITY

The passive person is generally characterized as quiet and shy and usually tends to withdraw from situations of any risk or conflict. This is the "wallflower" at parties, or the resentful employee who never asks for a raise, or the fat lady tugging at the folds of her muumuu, or the child who hangs onto Daddy's leg, peering meekly around the trouser to see without being seen. We have all felt this way at one time or another. Passive people often prejudge themselves and others, saying, "You're okay, I'm not okay."

Polly Passive is often admired, sometimes pitied, rarely invited, usually tolerated, and never envied. That is the bottom line and the essential reason to remain passive. It is also the rallying cry of many an E-D:

"I don't want to make anyone else feel bad. I'll be uncomfortable instead."

"I'm already so physically large, I want to minimize any other effects I'm having."

"I don't want anyone to feel uncomfortable around me."

Passivity can also be used as a way to subtly but powerfully control others. Polly Passive whines about how helpless she is so others will come in and do it for her. In that way, she never lives up to her own potential and is living in that dress rehearsal, waiting until, "I get strong enough . . . rich enough . . . thin enough. . . ." As long as she remains rigidly passive and someone else is the actor in her life, she hides in food. Her lament rings:

"I never seem to be able to accomplish anything."

"I sure wish I could help, but I'd mess it up."

"What can you expect from a fat person."

"Don't ask of me, I'm starving myself."

Passive behavior can be healthy and nurturing occasionally. Sometimes, it may be a strategic advantage to keep quiet instead of raising the roof. Withdrawal is sometimes actually more active than jumping in with both feet. When a passive mode becomes your only style, then it is self-destructive. You have limited options. You have to be passive when every instinct in your body is crying out for action. When you rigidly remain passive no matter what, you are going to have troubles when the body screams, "I wanna come out and dive into my life." Sometimes the only way you know to shut up the wailing inner self is to drown it out with food.

As a codependent to this person, you may not like the E-D's passivity. You don't have to. Remember, your job is to work your own side of the street. In the past you became more active to counter the passivity. Now you don't enjoy that role all the time. At your meetings you can fall apart. In taking care of yourself, you must state your needs. Instead of rescuing, you will be making more demands on the E-D. You must give up being the caretaker. If you are trying to take care of yourself and them at the same time, you will have too much conflict. Imagine the problem if you want to insure that the E-D feels satisfied, but what would satisfy them is something that makes you feel deprived. You both need petting at exactly the same time. You could end up like two-year-olds battling over toys in a playpen. At this point, it's better to seek your separate solutions with your individual sponsors.

AGGRESSION

Andy Aggressive hits others before they have a chance to hit him. Much of his energy is spent covering all bases so no one can criticize him for anything or take advantage of him. His tombstone will read, "Nobody got the best of him." His aggression stems from the same inadequate feelings as Polly Passive, but he found another way to cope with them. He strikes out with, "I'm okay, you're not!" He will do all he can to make you and himself believe that. He has to gorge himself to keep his true fear hidden. He loudly disclaims any vulnerable feelings, often using direct attack, personal ridicule, or subtle sarcasm:

"You'd better not try to take advantage of me."

"I'll make you pay for that."

"So, you think you're hot stuff, eh?"

"I like my belly. Doc told me to watch my weight, so I've got it out there where I can watch it—ha, ha, ha."

Aggression protects. The best defense is a good offense. Just as Polly used passivity as a subtle form of control, Andy uses aggressiveness as another. He does not want to show his vulnerability. If he looks tough and keeps you distant, either laughing or quivering, then he feels safe. How could anyone expect such a tough guy to be vulnerable? You buy his facade and leave him alone. His aggressive posture is really too much to take on. Others buy the act and leave. Without food, the aggression breaks down and the scared little boy comes out.

There are some aspects of aggressiveness that work for survival. Aggression helps you overcome fear and succeed in a competitive environment. You then mobilize the energy needed for difficult tasks. You will be warned when you are threatened. Some aggressive instinct is necessary. Without it, you'll be victimized all the time. You don't want to completely discard this aspect of yourself. Instead, you need to choose when and where to mobilize aggression. Make it work for you rather than against you.

ASSERTIVENESS

Ideally you will strive for a neutral position—neither passive nor aggressive. The assertive person mobilizes either passive or aggressive behavior as needed. Life has its ebb and flow and the assertive person has enough personal security to roll with the punches and adopt a style to fit the occasion. The assertive response to conflict is, "I'm okay and you're okay. If there is a problem between us we can work it out." As an assertive person, you watch out for your own best interests and make decisions accordingly. You might decide it is better not to defend some positions, and then take a stand on others which some people would let go by. You become your own judge, little motivated by what others want or expect. Pliant and flexible, you become truly natural and alive.

For detailed descriptions of assertive techniques, I recommend a book by psychologist Manuel J. Smith, Ph.D. Its title clearly highlights the lament of the E-D and codependent, *When I Say No, I Feel Guilty.*[1] You will learn ways of responding to guilt and criticism. Few of us need much help in responding to praise. We usually weather that fairly well. (Sometimes an E-D is excessively shy and can't take praise, and so responds to compliments with elaborate disclaimers.) To recover you must learn to weather criticism. Even if it isn't the other guy criticizing, your own judge sits on your shoulder and reads you the riot act. You need to learn an assertive response. This internal judge is with you all the time and works overtime to tell you when you are wrong. When you believe this judge, you can turn to food to punish yourself. The codependent turns to being more and more abusive of the E-D. You each end up guilty. There is a better way out. Let's see how to say no to our judge (whether internal or from outside) and instead say yes to life.

As you are a person in recovery, you learn new choices about where to focus your energies. You gain a new sense of priorities about the important issues in your life. Keeping abstinence first helps move the "judge" aside. "I may not be perfect, but at least I'm following my committed food plan. I will get better later. 'Progress, not perfection.' "

When you feel criticized, try to agree with the truthful part of the criticism. You do not have to buy the entire criticism; you just agree with the part of it that you find true. For example, when someone says, "You are really fat and ugly," you reply, "I am big, aren't I?" End of sentence, say no more. Just agree with the part you find to be true.

Sometimes you agree with the probability that what the other person is saying is correct. For example, you would use phrases

---

[1] Available through Hazelden Educational Materials, Box 176, Pleasant Valley Road, Center City, MN 55012.

such as, "You *may* be right," "That's *possibly* true," "*Odds are,* you are correct," or, "*Chances are,* that is so."

You also use this technique in response to criticism such as, "You always . . . ," or, "You never. . . ." For example:

They say	You reply
"You're gonna die if you keep eating like that!"	"You may be right."
"You never do the dishes."	"Sometimes I don't do the dishes."
"You probably weigh 300 pounds!"	"That could be true."
"You always embarrass me in public."	"Sometimes I have embarrassed you in public."

You have agreed. Don't disagree. Disagreeing only encourages argument. You have shown you don't wish to argue. That is assertive. You represent yourself without violating anyone else. There is no cause for guilt here and thus no cause for punishment. You will find this helpful when others are using scare tactics to get you to do things their way.

To cover over your own self-loathing, you often avoided saying no and were thus continually manipulated, and later angry. Your solution was food. Now you can find new ways to handle the con artist. People manipulate through phrases that start with *if.* These statements involve the other person's ideas of how they feel you should act.

"If you loved me, you'd bring me some candy."
"If you were a good friend, you'd loan me $500."
"If you cared, you'd stop my eating."
"If you valued your health, you'd diet."

In sorting the issues, separate the phrases. You may respond with

"I do love you, *and* I don't want to bring candy."
"I am a good friend, *and* I won't loan you $500."
"I do care, *and* I can't fix you."
"I *do* value my health, *and* dieting is not a good style for me."

Emphasize the "and." You show there is no relationship between the first and second statements. A loved one does not have to bring candy. You *can* value your health *and* not do it "their way."

It is important to use "and" rather than "but." When you say "but" you imply a relationship between point A and point B. When you say "and," you are clearly separating. Notice the difference.

"I really like you, *but* (hedging) I can't have dinner with you."

"I really do like you, *and* (definite) right now I'm not able to have dinner with you." (It also helps to say "right now" so later you have the option to change your mind.)

To maintain your own assertive position, you can remain interested in the opinions of others, but not dominated by them. It is a thin line. You can show that you are genuinely interested in hearing more from this person, but don't choose to be criticized.

You ask questions so they can refine their comments. Ask them to be specific and really itemize their particular objection or criticism. You want them to own their own criticisms.

They say	You reply
"When are you going to lose some weight?"	"I am not really clear about why you think I haven't been trying to lose weight. Can you explain more fully in what way you are disappointed?"

Do not ask this as a "come on" to argue, but rather with genuine concern. You want them to be clearer in owning their own judgments of you.

You want the person to directly state how they feel. You'd like them to move from making "you" statements to making "I" statements. Then you can take it or leave it. "Thanks for sharing that. Now, I understand your position."

"YOU MADE ME LOVE YOU"

Laments of "I couldn't help myself" are borrowed from Top-40 music charts and used by E-Ds to break their commitments to themselves. Although we believe keeping promises to others is gracious, we think keeping promises to ourselves is selfish. When you start seeing that your eating disorder is an illness rather than a morality issue, you will be able to say no as a part of your prescription for recovery.

Other people are used as excuses for slips in food commitments.

"They made me do it."

"It was Aunt Rebecca's favorite recipe."

"She'd be insulted."

"The whole family was celebrating Thanksgiving. How could I refuse?"

"Do you really think I would insult the bride by not having a piece of wedding cake?"

Let's face it. There is only one person at that whole wedding who gives a damn one way or the other whether you eat the cake or not. That is you. The bride has plenty of other things to occupy her time. The groom isn't going to think you wish them 40 years of bad luck. No one cares! But you do. It's your obsession talking you into eating. A committee holds a meeting in your head and starts talking you into "just one piece." Your committee is working overtime to talk you into it. You envision a giant spotlight shining on you while everyone in the room waits in hushed anticipation to see which way you will go with the cake. All you need is for one well-meaning, sympathetic friend to say, "Go ahead. It's a special occasion and it's only one piece."

"Well, geez Ma, the devil made me do it." In reality, it is your obsessive love affair with food that makes you do it. You only use others to talk you into what the sick side of you had already planned. "Well, everyone else was having some. It's not fair! Why me?" (Anger and denial.) Others at the wedding who aren't E-Ds will eat one piece and forget it. You will have one piece, then a few bites off a friend's plate when they aren't looking, then a small fingerful of icing when Janet pushes hers away, declaring, "It's just too sweet for me." Later that night you wonder what happened to the rest of that big cake. You think maybe you should have taken a piece home. The cake drama doesn't stop at bedtime. The next day finds you barrelling down a supermarket aisle tearing open cellophane bags of malted milk balls trying to recapture yesterday's sweetness.

There is a way out of this scenario. You need to put just as much energy into a new response as you previously put into bingeing.

You have to see abstinence as a reward rather than a deprivation. The reward will be that you are available to feel and live your own life. Let's see how Denise gave herself a gift by not having the cake at her sister's wedding. Her Aunt Ann was the most forceful "pusher" at the party. Denise gave herself the gift of abstinence while Aunt Ann was slicing.

Ann: Here Denise, have a piece and wish your sister luck.

Denise: No thank you, Aunt Ann.

Ann: Come on, Denise, this is no time to be on a diet. (Notice Denise's refusal of the cake was not followed by "I'm on a diet." There's no need to say that. If we do, we set it up for others to try to talk us into breaking a diet. Never say diet! Notice how normal people don't make big shows of explaining the whats and whys of their eating. They simply say, "No thanks.")

Denise: No thanks. I'm not on a diet. I just don't care for any right now. (Notice how Denise repeats the "no" for herself as much as for Ann—it's reinforcing. She also says, no for now, which implies she may have some later. Sometimes that can put off someone who is "pushing." It didn't stop Aunt Ann.)

Ann: What's the matter, Denise? Are you resentful and jealous that your sister is getting married before you? Here come the criticisms! These questions appear well-meaning, as if the inquisitor is really interested. In reality, it is a very cheap shot cloaked in cliches implying sibling rivalry and all that "psychobabble." If Aunt Ann is really interested in what you are feeling, she is not going to ask such an intimate question over a buffet table while slicing wedding cake. She really doesn't want an answer; she wants to let you know she's got your number. This type of interchange is a violation. A quick easy response is to pick up the cake and stuff it in to keep your mouth shut. In such a scenario, your head says, "These are loving, nurturing people with your best interests at heart." Your body feels stab wounds all over your chest. If you feel wounded, it's because you have been. Remember, the body doesn't lie. Don't eat the cake, feel the pain.

Denise: Actually, Ann, I don't think that's it. Thanks anyway. (Denise answers enough to the criticism by saying she doesn't agree. She'll judge her own behavior, thank you. She also does not offer any further explanation or argument.)

Ann: (relentless) Well, if I were you, I'd take a look at my real feelings about this wedding. (Again, a criticism. "Auntie knows best. You don't even know your 'real' feelings. I have to interpret for you.")

Denise: Thanks for your concern, and no thanks to the cake.

CASE CLOSED.

Denise offers no explanations, and gives Ann the benefit of the doubt. Maybe her comments are out of concern, and she doesn't notice how violating she is. Denise got out alive without overexplaining herself, and, most importantly, without eating the cake. During this interchange, Denise secretly cheered herself on, "No matter what, this bitch won't make me eat." She had to overcome a very strong power struggle. Refusing the cake left her exhilarated. Her strength and confidence lasted through the afternoon and well into the night. The cake didn't dominate her thoughts, self-respect did. She knew she was terrific. She felt so good that, later at the party, she walked up to a good looking, unattached man and asked him to dance. She'd never done anything like that in her life! Incapacitated with shyness, her usual mode was to linger around buffet tables, bingeing, as a way to ignore the shyness trauma.

Instead, she felt "high" and deserving, because she refused the cake. Saying no to food made her more committed to saying yes to life. When not eating compulsively, there is much more impetus to "go for it." Why not? We deserve it all! The good looking man took her phone number. She spent that evening very pleased with herself for resisting the cake and Aunt Ann, and dreamily contemplating her new relationship. Without shutting herself up with food, Denise found an outgoing, risky woman inside. What a surprise!

"AREN'T YOU GETTING TOO DEPENDENT?"

Annabelle, a diabetic, was referred to me by an internist. When we met, she was highly deferential, extolling the virtues of Dr. Atwell.

"He has been our family physician for years. He really knows his stuff. If he says I should get involved in this recovery program, I'm certainly ready!" Unfortunately, at that point, Dr. Atwell knew very little about the newly-instituted hospital program for eating disorders. He just knew how many physicians' efforts had failed with Annabelle. She responded to doctors' orders in a fairly typical way. She giggled shyly and, with wide-eyed charm, promised the doctor that she really valued his advice and would follow his suggestions. She'd leave the office embarrassed about her apparent lack of willpower. As the nurse gave a few "tsks, tsks" while she weighed Annabelle, she was humiliated by her own giggly behavior around powerful people. The situation was so demeaning that she heightened her self-loathing by "kissing up" to the professional. Her giggles and posing helped mask her rage at even having to visit the doctor's office.

She came to me with the same "tell me what to do" attitude. Her recovery was ultimately secured when she learned to tell professionals she didn't need them to tell her what to do. Her past behavior had shown she didn't follow doctors' orders anyway. She needed to find a way to say no out loud. Her chance came three months after her initial referral. She had been abstinent from compulsive eating and refined carbohydrates for 76 days. She had a brief relapse one weekend, but got back on her program quickly and lost 41 pounds! Best of all, her blood-sugar level and blood pressure had normalized. This woman had previously required daily insulin injections. She knew that eating sugar was deadly for her, but kept bingeing periodically. As an E-D, she can't control herself without help. At each of her weekly checkups, Dr. Atwell was more and more impressed with how well she was doing. Rather than passively waiting for him or the nurse to deliver her a lecture, Annabelle took control of the visits. She talked animatedly about how well she was doing at Overeaters Anonymous. She got excited sharing with them how much fun the meetings were and how much support she was getting from her sponsor. She elaborated on how she managed to survive a family dinner party without bingeing and was looking forward to throwing away her injection syringes. This was a threat to Dr. Atwell.

At this juncture, Annabelle was changing the rules and the roles. SHE was telling the physician what SHE had planned in her recovery program. Understandably, he became medically concerned, as he was "responsible" and, of course, had seen her relapse before. It was hard for him to believe this time will be different. He wanted more control of the situation.

Dr. Atwell: Well, Annabelle, it does seem like you are well on the road. We will want to keep monitoring you weekly just to make sure you have no problems. (Dr. Atwell was trying to continue the same old relationship. The physician will ultimately be in control, and Annabelle will passively reject his advice.)

Annabelle: Actually, Dr. Atwell, I don't think I should see you every week. It is better for me to only weigh in once a month. You see, I have a tendency to become obsessed with the scale and it's best if I just stay abstinent in my eating rather than looking forward to weighing. (Annabelle made more explanation here than necessary, but this was because she was trying to educate the doctor about the needs of others like herself. This was definitely a role reversal and threat to their relationship. Dr. Atwell was accustomed to passive, guilty patients. Annabelle was taking too much control over her own recovery. The doctor was concerned for her as she "might relapse" and also somewhat disgruntled at her telling him how it's gonna be.)

Dr. Atwell: You know Annabelle, you do have a tendency to fall back on your commitments. I think we better continue a closer watch on you. (Staying with the past.)

Annabelle: I understand your concern (active listening: letting him know she heard and understood him), *and* I am finding that daily contact with others in Overeaters Anonymous is helping me stay abstinent. (Sorting issues.)

Dr. Atwell: Yes, but you do need a close watch so we can detect any blood-sugar fluctuations. (The doctor wanted to turn the discussion to areas of his expertise so he could feel more in control and move Annabelle to her usual "one-down" position.)

Annabelle: I have been abstinent from sugars long enough that my body is becoming a very sensitive barometer. Since

I talk daily with someone else about my eating, I think we would see a problem long before it would show up on lab tests. I'd rather head my eating off in advance than dissect my blood after the fact.

This turn of events can be very disconcerting to medical personnel. A patient who has been chronically obese, and diabetic, spending countless hours in physician's waiting rooms, is telling her doctor she would rather go to meetings with lay people and seek their help rather than his professional services! Professionally concerned for the patient's health, the doctor returns to what he knows best as medical technique. He wants to be more cautious and keep control of the situation. Unconsciously, the doctor is personally threatened by this new development. He is concerned that a group of nonprofessionals accomplish what has stymied him for years. It is the rare professional who can let the patient go find her own best recovery. The doctor must be secure that he has already done all he can and will be willing to let others try. In this case, it was clear that Annabelle was definitely committed to taking over responsibility for her own recovery. This was a dramatic change from the doctor-patient relationship they had had for the past twenty years.

Dr. Atwell did make one last attempt to turn her around. He saw that Annabelle's attendance at O.A. was definitely accomplishing what had stymied him in the past. He knew it was working. He congratulated her on her progress each time she came to his office. Despite all the indications that this was the way to go, he still doubted its validity. He was concerned that Annabelle said she had a lifelong, chronic illness and would always need to rely on some type of help. (This was not a problem for him if the help required was from a physician. He was concerned that Annabelle was accepting the idea that she'd need to rely on other suffering E-Ds!)

He made one more attempt to warn Annabelle about the dangers of diminishing her visits. "Don't you think you've had enough of those meetings? Do you want to go to them for *the rest of your life?* It's just another dependency."

Annabelle smiled, "You *may* be right. I try to take my recovery 'one day at a time.' For *now,* this seems to be what I need. I'd like to follow through with this just for today. I like the idea that 'if it works, don't fix it.'"

Dr. Atwell stared blankly. What could he say? He can't argue with results. In taking responsibility for her own recovery and going for help where she was equal rather than subordinate, Annabelle started actively participating in her life. As she became more successful in her food plan, she felt more secure and assertive.

Dr. Atwell's concerns bring up a commonly voiced criticism of successful members of Overeaters Anonymous. While they are still fat, no one criticizes their attendance at meetings, but after most of the weight is lost, others start doubting the necessity for attendance. "Don't you think you've been going to those meetings long enough? You've lost your weight. Don't you think you could cut down now? After all, you don't want to develop *dependency.*" This thinking is puzzling. Wasn't the obsessive addiction to bingeing a dependency? Aren't many in our culture dependent on other drugs and obsessions? What is wrong with transferring the dependency to something healthy and nurturing? It's not such a terrible thing to admit that, "Yes, I am a person who likes supportive, loving people, and when I go to meetings I feel nurtured and don't have to go home and binge." What is wrong with depending on love? Our little dog at home doesn't consider all this when he rolls over to be petted. Why are humans so afraid to get love? A person with a broken leg would be foolish to refuse setting the bone in a cast and walking with crutches. Can't a sick and suffering E-D turn to others who can help heal and support? Why not? So you need a crutch. . . .

Critics who tell E-Ds not to go to O.A. are trying to live by the American macho myth: "I can do it myself." Even if you could, why *should* you?

WHAT'S YOUR FORTUNE, COOKIE?

As a codependent, you must learn to stand up for your own feelings around the E-D. You have spent so long developing a chameleon-like ability to "walk in their shoes" and adjust to their moods, that it is hard for you to learn that how *you* feel is important. *How you feel* does not have to be explained, justified, or excused. It just is. Emotions are not right or wrong. They just are. Your hardest job is learning to take care of yourself, not them.

Roberta got a chance to test out her new assertive skills when she took her overeating daughter, Claire, out to lunch. Claire had come home on a pass from the treatment unit, and asked her mom to take her to lunch. "I'm just dying for some Chinese food! Let's go to Foo Long's."

As soon as these words were out, Roberta began to panic. She saw Claire's eyes light up. Roberta knew she didn't want to take responsibility for Claire's food plan, that it was not her business how Claire ate, but she felt sick inside. It was the glow, that look! Family members can see that haze reappear when a binge is imminent. Claire looked like a convict, just released, ready to commit another crime. Roberta didn't want any part of it. She tried to respond by expressing her own feelings rather than telling Claire how to act or feel.

Roberta: Honey, I don't feel comfortable going to that restaurant.

Claire: Oh, wow, mom. You're trying to control my food again. If you weren't so controlling, we'd go there.

Roberta: It's not control. I just don't want to be there today.

Claire: Would you want to go if it was someone else rather than me?

Roberta: (Self-disclosure must be the truth.) Well, yes.

Claire: (attacking) See! It's just that you want to keep me from eating Chinese food.

Roberta: I am not concerned with what you eat. That is your business.

Claire: (escalating) That's right. I'll eat what I want, when I want, and I don't have to take orders from you! If you'd stop controlling, we'd go there.

Roberta: I don't want to control *and* I don't want to go to Foo Long's today (sticking to "I" messages). I don't want to give you any orders.

Claire: Then, why won't you go to Foo Long's with me?

Roberta: (She *asked* so it's not "butting in" to answer. Roberta sticks with "I" messages about her own feelings.) Well Dear, since you asked, I will share with you how it is for me. It is hard for me to be with you when I sense this panicked, ravenous feeling about food. It makes me feel bad to watch you. I feel that when you are in the midst of that, it's better we be apart. I love to eat with you when you are in a calmer state about food.

Claire: (Her mother's honest statement of her own feelings helped Claire to really hear what was said. This let her open up to look at herself.) Do I really seem ravenous? I thought I just wanted to return there for old time's sake. I didn't even know.

Roberta: We've been there often during binge times, and it may just be my memories, but I'd rather not go there right now. (Notice Roberta states 'just for today.' This is how she feels about it today. It may not be for all time. She just has to express where she is today.) I do feel a little anxiety from you. Like, it's really so important to make it that place. I'm just uncomfortable.

Claire: Now that you mention it, I think I'm uncomfortable too. I really noticed myself getting excited about Foo Long's. Come to think of it, I was really kind of obsessing about their sweet and sour pork. I felt like I had it coming to me.

Roberta: I guess that's what I picked up, that excitement.

Claire: I really don't want to eat anything that is calling to me that much. I can only eat it if I can take it or leave it. If I've got to have it, I can't.

Roberta: Well, Sweetheart, your food is your business. I just had to tell you that I felt too much anxiety to go there today.

Claire: Thanks Mom. Wanna go to the coffee shop where they make that nice salmon?

TRADING ROLES FOR REALITIES

Sometimes one person is both an eating disorder sufferer and codependent, and attends both Overeaters Anonymous and O-Anon. Many couples are both E-D and codependent. It is very easy to begin comparing, competing, and evaluating your partner's recovery instead of your own. You need to find a positive way to tell your mate to mind his or her own business. Racine and Joe had to work this out after Racine met a friend for dinner at a salad bar restaurant.

Joe: Racine, since I've been in the recovery program, I've been advised that it's not a good idea to go out to salad bar restaurants. (Joe is trying to come across as assertive, but underneath, he is implying that "father knows best" and "you'd better listen to me.")

Racine: Oh? (She knows he wants her to change her behavior and do it "his way," but she doesn't react. She waits. Her response is a form of negative inquiry. She is asking him to provide more information to get to the point of what he really wants to say.)

Joe: Yes, Dear. I don't think you should go to that salad bar much.

Racine: I see. How does that affect you Joe? (Racine is trying to get Joe to make an "I" statement and stop telling her what to do with her life.)

Joe: Well, I've been watching and I really think you are packing in more food than you need. You don't notice yourself at salad bars.

Racine: And how does that affect you, Joe?

Joe: Well, it really doesn't affect me at all. I'm just telling you for your own good. Take it or leave it. (Joe is becoming defensive because he is being asked to *own* his own feelings and be more direct and assertive. He'd rather tell her what to do than state how he feels. He could have made an "I" statement by saying, "I don't like it!" That might be too risky for him at this point.)

Racine: (Letting him know that she is feeling secure with her own food plan.) I hear your concerns, *and* I feel I am getting enough help with my food plan. My sponsor and I feel the salad bar fits in well. (This is END OF REPORT. Racine has let Joe know that she will be a person who judges her own behavior, and she will not need to explain herself to anyone. Since she is also working actively with her sponsor in O.A., she can feel secure that her food plan is organized, disciplined, and healthy, and that she isn't kidding herself about her eating. Security about the food creates security in interpersonal relating.)

SELF-DISCLOSURE

It is ideal to be able to express your own feelings and thoughts to another *without hurting them or yourself.* This depends on the nature of your relationship and how strongly you feel about yourself and your position.

It is important that you make "I" statements about yourself and your feelings rather than "you" statements about the other person. You are best at representing yourself and how *you* feel.

Example: "I am hurt by your criticism."
           "I really wish I felt more liked by you."
           "I'm afraid you don't like me."
           "I'm afraid you might leave me."
           "I feel badly at disappointing you."
           "I am embarrassed by my fat."
           "I feel a lot of pressure when you ask my weight."

Rita had been anorexic and her mom was grateful she was finally eating again. However, Mom wanted to move their relating away from food. They were always discussing food and diet. Mom lamented, "Is this all there is?" She wanted more. Her sponsor in O-Anon helped her learn a more assertive response to Rita.

Rita: (calling on telephone) Hi Mom, how about dinner next week?
Mom: Well, Rita, I'd love to see you, and I'd rather not go to dinner.
Rita: What do you mean? You have to eat don't you?
Mom: Yes.
Rita: Well, why not with me? Don't you want me to eat?
Mom: It's up to you if you eat or not. Whatever you like. I'd just rather do something else.
Rita: I get it. You're trying to control my food again.
Mom: I miss having other experiences that don't center on eating or not eating. For me, it gets in the way. I'd rather do other things with you. Truthfully, I do tend to watch what you eat an awful lot. I get overly concerned when you pick at your food. I watch how you 'work your plate.' I think it interferes with our relationship. I'd like to do something with you that has nothing to do with food. Let's see what else we have going for us.

Mom remained secure with her own "I" messages about what "I" would like. She did not respond to Rita's invitation to fight about control. She is saying she would like to see Rita, that she cares, and that she is *owning* her own tendency to want to control. She is also opening up to the idea that food is getting in the way and she wants to be close to Rita instead. She's tired of hovering over her daughter's plate.

In this case, even though Mom did very well in being direct and stating her own wishes, Rita was really looking for a binge buddy. The best binge buddy is often a punitive parent. They join in and then punish. With that you can have it both ways. Unfortunately, this mom didn't want that role anymore, and Rita wasn't ready to stop the game.

Rita: (Angrily) Well, I think it's just you trying to make me eat your way again. If you weren't such a control freak, you could stand to watch me eat whatever and however I want. You are letting your problem with my eating get in the way. (Actually this is improvement for Rita. In the past she never expressed rage. A benchmark book on anorexia is titled, *The Best Little Girl in the World*. She was always a "good girl" while starving herself.)

Mom: (Agreeing with the odds) You may be right, *and* rather than test myself or you, I'd rather move our relationship to another arena. I'd like to go to the museum.

Rita: Too bad, Mom. If you can't accept me as I am, eating as I do, then I want nothing more to do with you.

Mom: You seem to be angry with me. I'm sorry you feel that way. Please do understand that I really would like to go to the museum, or a street fair, or crafts show, or anything else you might like. Please let me know if you'd like to try something like that. (Mom continues with "I" messages despite the attack. She doesn't let her agenda be swayed by Rita's anger.)

Both of these women are changing their old roles with each other. For today, they are able to stand separately and express themselves. This interchange highlights a crucial issue in eating relationships.

Maybe Rita and her mom have nothing in common other than their power struggles over food. When one person withdraws from that struggle, there may be nothing left. They deserve the chance to find out.

"BEAT ME, BABY!"

Many obese women beg their passive husbands to be stronger with them. Often, the husband is really not too interested in interacting anyway, and even if he has tried, can't seem to match his wife's intensity. He may retreat into a passive acceptance of their situation. Sometimes the passivity comes out in sideline aggression rather than direct frontal attack.

Elizabeth had been after Joel for years, demanding that he stand up to her. She complained that she felt spoiled and out of control and wanted him to set limits for her. This is part of the E-D's wish to stay childlike, but in control. Joel was a former truck driver. He had dislocated a hip in an accident and was now permanently retired. He also suffered a hearing loss and counted on Elizabeth to be his ears. He rarely went anywhere without Elizabeth and never asked others to speak up. It was easier to have Elizabeth translate. In exchange for this, Joel was Elizabeth's servant. She weighed over 400 pounds and found it difficult to walk or breathe. Joel answered her every need. He picked up her dropped pencils, prepared her meals, buttoned her clothes, even helped her out of low-slung chairs. They functioned well together as invalids. As their relationship became more and more dependent, neither left home much. He cooked, she ate.

Recovery was a definite threat to that self-enclosed system. Joel secretly feared for Elizabeth's health, suspecting an imminent heart attack; he was also, frankly, tired of picking up after her. Like many spouses of chronically ill and addicted people, he suffered too, and felt both grief and anger at the same time. The codependent has compassion for the suffering of the addicted person, but also feels helpless watching him or her slowly deteriorate. He feels enraged by his own inability to help. Joel even admitted he would prefer Elizabeth end it all quickly rather than to watch the daily trauma of her slow suicide. Joel felt it was inappropriate for him to feel anger toward a sick person. He was frustrated because he had no emotional outlets. Elizabeth often asked him to express himself, but actually feared he would. She knew he was angry. His behavior let her know. But he never said anything directly. There was too much to lose.

Joel had to confront his own denial. He began saying no to

her. He sat tight while he watched her struggle to pick up a pencil. Stopping old, predictable behaviors is another way of saying no. Actions speak louder than words. Elizabeth had never had to suffer the consequences of her disorder. Joel was always there to rescue her. She occupied a PIP, or Priviledged Invalid Position, in the family. Elizabeth actually felt she deserved special services from Joel because she had worked hard raising his two children from a previous marriage. Although she did deserve to be treated well, their arrangement was killing her!

After a few weeks in O-Anon, Joel became more assertive with Elizabeth and told her, lovingly, that he would not be her servant anymore. No one likes to be told no, and Elizabeth was no exception. She attacked Joel, accusing him of neglect. Joel had worked hard to suppress his anger for many years and found it hard to fight back. He found his strength in a family therapy session with the support of other codependents. He finally summoned the courage to answer back. He stood up and with quivering jaw and stern look shouted, "Dammit, woman, either respect me or leave me!" The room echoed with silence. Elizabeth was stunned, then beamed with respect. She cried, "I'll never say another mean thing to you again." She feared he would really leave her if things didn't change. She was scared. He had options. She marvelled at the realization that he was a separate person. She also knew he meant what he said. He had support from other codependents and didn't feel guilty. He learned that her recovery was her job. He had never been that strong with her before, and *she loved it.* For years she had whined at him to be stronger. Each time he was it was meaningless because she had asked for it. This time it was totally his idea. Neither one of them has forgotten that night. It signalled the beginning of a new life; no going back and nowhere to hide.

As a way of pretending she didn't mind her Priviledged Invalid Position, Elizabeth often made fun of herself and played the clown. This way she stayed in control; she made fun of herself before anyone else could. Whenever she huffed and puffed into a room, she quipped, "I'm such a tub o' lard, I hope I don't break this chair! Ha, ha, ha." Ridiculing herself was a meaningless way to pay Joel back for all he'd done for her. She had so dehumanized herself (to a "tub") that she never respected her own feelings. When Joel broke through his own fear of anger, she was forced to take herself more seriously. If he could demand respect, so could she.

Elizabeth learned to see herself as a suffering person trying to get well and started respecting herself. She began to talk at O.A. meetings and share the pain of her obesity. She had to get close with strangers first before she could come closer to Joel. She had to hear herself say, "I feel really badly about my weight, and I'm tired of making jokes about myself." Today, both she and Joel attend separate meetings where they can talk about their own separate feelings; then, when they come together, they're both more assertive.

A year and 200 lost pounds later, I asked them, "What if someone said that recovery has made you and Joel distant from each other? You used to be together every minute. Now you go to separate meetings and you argue more than you used to." Both were incredulous at the idea. Joel explained the new freedom he feels at not being under the gun or managed by Elizabeth's dependency. "She's got her problems, I've got mine."

Elizabeth smiled coquettishly. "Since we've developed our separate identities, our sex life is coming back, and that's great!"

It's not as much fun to have sex with yourself as with a partner. Developing their separateness helped them come together in a much more exciting way.

When I met with them after the first year, we were seated in low, engulfing overstuffed chairs in the hospital lounge. Elizabeth asked Joel to bring her two straight chairs to use as support to help her up. There were only folding chairs. She looked around and then wondered aloud if they were strong enough to help her to stand. Looking at Joel, the chairs and then me she said, "Oh, the hell with it. I'll do it myself." A deep breath, a slight sigh, a push and Elizabeth was out of the chair. Joel beamed his approval. He had worked himself out of the job!

HEALTHY NEUTRALITY

With new assertiveness, you won't have to force your ideas on each other, and you'll learn to mind your own business. As you attend your own self-help groups, you will be too busy to monitor anyone else. Getting your own house in order is a full-time job. Each of you deserve the support and nurturance of others. And you deserve to feel good about the love you give someone else. It is surely difficult when you do your best and give your all, and the one you love and care for is still miserable and hurting. It is very hard to give up the job of "helping" them. However, that often proves to be the most loving thing you can do. By removing yourself from your loved one's struggle, you help them get help from someone else. That doesn't make you inadequate; it just means the job was not yours to take on. Perhaps you are too close and they love you too much. In their zeal to please you, they may not be able to find the path to their own recovery. It is difficult to see that letting go is helpful.

Again, we confront the message, LOSE TO WIN. You are working toward developing a new loving relationship with an equal, not tackling a "project." If you wanted the job of battling illness, you should have become a doctor. It is good to separate the person from the disease. You may continue to love the person but you do not have to enjoy the sickness.

Once you have mastered a healthy neutrality toward one another, you will undoubtedly encounter the usual struggles others have when an eating disorder is not in the picture. In any relationship, despite whatever good will exists, conflicts occur. One wants to go to the show and the other wants to stay home. One wants to wallpaper the living room and the other thinks plaster is best. Both want to use the car on the same night. Each is in a bad mood on the same day.

Even knowing the proper responses as outlined in this chapter won't help if your tone and attitude still hark back to the past. That is why the self-help groups of O.A. and O-Anon are so important. Others can see your attitudes better than you can. They can give you feedback about how you are really coming across. They will interpret your nonverbal messages and help you hear what you're not saying. The meetings will be your practice field, so you can come back to the relationship and play "the best game in town."

Even before you begin to use your groups for practice, it is helpful to keep the following guidelines as a clue for yourself. The suggested DOs and DON'Ts can be followed by both E-Ds and codependents as you are both fellow victims of eating disorders. You will both have a tendency to relapse into past behaviors, the E-D bingeing and the codependent obsessing about watching. If recovery lasts a lifetime, there is bound to be periodic relapse which you should try not to judge, but wait through, and then go on. Try to realize that when there is relapse, the one suffering is hurting themselves, not trying to hurt you. They are not doing it to you. They are just doing it. Take care of yourself and work your own side of the street.

DOs AND DON'Ts FOR E-Ds AND CODEPENDENTS

DON'T preach and lecture to your wife, husband, parent, child, etc.

DON'T have a "holier-than-thou" attitude.

DON'T use the "if you loved me" appeal.

DON'T make threats you won't carry out.

DON'T scold about the past.

DON'T hide food or avoid social engagements.

DON'T argue when bingeing.

DON'T make an issue over treatment.

DON'T assume martyr-like self-pity.

DON'T expect an immediate, 100% recovery.

DON'T be jealous of the recovery.

DON'T be a doormat to the mood swings.

DON'T try to protect.

DON'T push anyone but yourself.

DO forgive.

DO learn the facts about eating disorders.

DO develop an attitude to match those facts.

DO talk to someone who *understands* (counselor, sponsor).

DO take a personal inventory of yourself and your behavior.

DO go to a clinic, treatment center, O-Anon or Al-Anon.

DO maintain a healthy atmosphere in the home.

DO encourage new interests, but don't nag.

DO take a relapse lightly if there is one.

DO pass on your knowledge to others.

DO be honest with yourself.

DO mind your own business.

DO take care of yourself.

DO try to relax and take it easy.

DO play—show you want a way out.

SUMMARY

Most of these techniques involve new behaviors which feel awkward at first. Give yourself a chance to be a beginner and a student.

You will need practice. First try it with a buddy from O.A. or O-Anon. Then, when you are more confident, bring them home to roost. Home is the most difficult battlefield, so practice with your extended family first.

You must pay careful attention to the effect you create with the other person. Obviously, it is easier to be strong and state your case with someone who is not a near and dear loved one. Practice assertiveness first with distant people, even strangers, and then move to directness with those you love. You don't want to wound the other person, either in the ego or the heart. You want to leave the situation feeling good about your own behavior and liking how you acted. You want to be able to look back at the situation and see yourself in action and say, "I really like how I handled that." When you feel good about how you behave with others, neither dominating nor being dominated, then you can relax and admire yourself. You won't have to punish yourself with food.

Chapter Eight

Fear of Flying

"This is it! It's my life. Whatever it takes, I want to spend the rest of it thinking about something other than food." Of course that's what you want. Then why have you spent the past 30, 40, or 50 years in the throes of the illness, denying what was happening to you while you sank lower into the suffering every day? Because you were afraid of flying! You didn't believe you deserved the good life.

We must believe that people respond appropriately, and that they do things for good reason. You had good reason to stay suffering with your eating disorder. One, of course, is because you didn't know. But now you've read this book. You chose to suffer rather than accept the alternative. The alternative would be life without pain and guilt. Many are afraid to be truly happy. You might feel too reckless and hedonistic. Many fear they'll be irresponsible and shallow if not suffering. Dragging around the excess suffering is a way to symbolically announce to the world that you care and are involved with its woes. So many popular public causes, whether banning bombs, helping poor, eliminating hunger, or saving whales, find their ranks swelling with bingers who demonstrate how much they care for others as a way to not appear self-involved and caring for *self*. If nothing else, this book is about learning to care for yourself before saving the world. Understandably, your new commitment to self might not be welcomed quickly by your fellow marchers who have come to depend on you for certain services. They may turn out to be the codependents who need to keep you in the same old role.

As an alternative to bingeing, you may find yourself going for weekly massages, manicures, or lunches with friends; activities you previously judged as too self-indulgent when there was so much important work to be done. For now, the most important work is to do whatever it takes to keep yourself serene and secure so you won't need to binge. Abstinence from the compulsion has to become your number one priority. Let yourself become a fanatic for your own cause.

There is a larger issue at hand here than just losing weight or getting a manicure. To truly gain a lifelong recovery, you will be renegotiating a basic commitment to yourself about your whole life. Are you ready and willing to become a person who actively responds to the good things in life? The suffering is always easy to find and you know how to react to it. The smooth comfortable old shoe of pain fits. How can you learn to endure your blessings?

If this were not a crucial aspect of recovery, we would not see so many people falling back into the throes of their illnesses. If you could handle the good life you certainly would not have picked up this book. You would not have gone back so many times. In this last chapter you will take a look at the imminent possibilities for your new life. You will see fears of success and how they relate to separating from home. Having been reparented in O.A. and O-Anon, you'll now have the security, encouragement, and self-worth to *go for it!*

FEAR OF SUCCESS

In a 100-mile journey, 90 is halfway. It's also true that the last ten pounds is often the killer for those overeaters who can't stand success. Of all Americans who undergo weight loss programs, after two years 97 percent gain all their weight back plus more! Even for those who have lost hundreds of pounds, the responsibilities of success seem to weigh them down again. If you've been one of these yo-yo dieters, you've witnessed this disappointment time and time again. The first few years, all the accolades and compliments seem to increase incentive and keep you committed. However, eventually applause for weight loss recedes and the world starts expecting more and different things from you. How do you live as an average Joe instead of a freak? While all were impressed with your success you were able to revel in the attention. At the same time, you feared they would go away. You anticipated taking on even greater challenges to make sure you maintained the attention.

Sometimes, that attention itself is aggravating. A dieter's body is public domain. Just the fact that the world comments about it makes it everyone else's province rather than your own. "Well, hi there skinny," someone says. "You're really losing weight!" You smile meekly and thank her, but a part of you feels violated. You don't comment on her body! It seems to be her own business. You want the compliment, you like being noticed. At the same time, it's a slight attack. It opens you to the possibility later that they'll readily comment if they see you gaining weight. You live in fear. What business is it of theirs?

You may have held the fat person's unrealistic sense of what the thin life is like. By imagining life will be perfect as soon as you lose weight, you face a number of disappointments and realities when you lose weight and still have normal human problems. You may decide you'd rather regain the weight and have that as your problem. At least that you know how to deal with. Returning to the starting gate in the weight loss race is easier; you know how to run that one. In other words, you won't have to learn any new tools or techniques for how to be a thin, "normal" person. If not diets, what else will you have to talk about? Even patients who lose hundreds of pounds with bypass surgery find that after two years, the pounds creep back on. At these wonders to medical science, the surgeon balks, "It's not possible that you can gain so much weight." He doesn't understand that you have to gain the weight or else face the harsher reality that you don't know how to live with the success you've always wanted. In my office hangs a picture poster showing a bright newly hatched yellow chick staring into space asking, "What do I do now?" That's the dieter's dilemma. The answer is, *stick with the winners.*

If you spent all these years in suffering, it is going to be hard to adjust and each day accept the good life. You will need to seek out and stay close to other successful people who will be happy for your success and not feel threatened. If you expand your circle of friends to include people who themselves are successful, they can teach you how to tolerate success and will also have no need to pull you back to old failures. (You'll get the nudge to "go for it" as you keep going to O.A.) Your success will only enhance and motivate them. They will have no need to see you fail, but will instead motivate and encourage you. Some meetings of Overeaters Anonymous are specifically designated as "maintainer's" meetings where success is the order of business. Discussions at these meetings center around living through the "stress of success" and "problems of abundance." Members need help to endure the good life. Let's look at some of the struggles with success voiced by effective maintainers. See if any of these statements could be voiced by you.

Equality

"I don't know how to deal with equality. I'm used to being with people I feel better than or less than. I don't know how to have an equal relationship. I walk on eggshells fearing you can't handle my strength. I don't want to talk much about when I am happy in case you don't feel the same way."

Loneliness

"I've done so well, why do I feel so bad? Things are great, but I feel lonely. Many of my old friends don't want to be with me anymore."

Friendships

"Without you I'm nothing, but with you I lose my sense of identity. When I'm not complaining about problems, I have very little to talk about."

Dependency

"I have to destroy myself and be needy in order to survive in a relationship. When I am not needy, nobody wants me."

Emotions

"I need to express my feelings, but I must be careful not to upset anyone. I have to balance on a tightrope—honest, but not too honest."

Differing Opinions

"If I don't see things as you do, I must be wrong. It's hard for me to believe I could be right. Does that make me wrong?"

Conflicts

"I have to learn to resolve differences without taking issues head on and embarrassing anyone. I've got to make others feel better."

Guilt

"I feel responsible for everyone's feelings, and at the same time, I don't have a clue what to do about their pain."

Myths

"I was taught to strive for success, but it's a hollow victory. Even when I'm a winner, I feel like a loser."

Models

"I don't know who to emulate. It seems like no one has trod this ground before me. No one I know is living how I'd like to live."

Health

"It's not so bad to get sick. Then I don't threaten anyone. I can get some nurturance without risk. If not weight problems, a migraine will suffice."

Sexuality

"But men don't like women like me. If I'm different, no one will want me."

Fears

"I want to try weird new things, but no one would even understand that I might like to. Where do I talk?"

Few have been given effective models for living with success. These models are provided at O.A. meetings by others further along in recovery. It is senseless to talk to them until you are approaching a stage closer to theirs. To the newcomer's explanation of being "afraid to get thin," the sponsor replied, "Well, get thin first and then we'll talk about it." In other words, it is not effective to examine these struggles until you are actually living with them. That is why O.A. is suggested as a lifelong support group. You will get what you need when you have gotten that much further on the path. You must avoid intellectualizing and philosophizing before you get there.

Opposite the hatched chick poster in my office is the midwifery diploma of my grandmother, Lena Glickfield Blumenfeld, issued in Vienna in 1905. I believe she helped people be born physically and, introducing E-Ds to O.A., I help them become reborn psychologically. In this new birth, you will be finding a way to tolerate success and avoid returning to past failure. You've already lived and died a thousand deaths. Your little chick never learned how to live. This time you'll be born with wings.

GROWING UP

The fear of moving along to success and accepting the joy in store stems from a deeper fear of growing up and leaving home. If you really stop being a suffering person and begin to take care of yourself in O.A. and in your life, it is a statement that you will be responsible for your own life and are giving up patterns you learned as a child. Often the codependent, whether it is your actual mother, a spouse you married who is like your mother, or a helpful friend who protects you like a mom, will have to find another job once the E-D is in recovery. As you become willing to do whatever it takes not to eat compulsively, then you are abandoning old patterns.

It is no accident that we see an epidemic of eating disorders in an age when youngsters are given so many conflicting messages about growing up to be responsible and at the same time remaining dependent and irresponsible. Eating disorders are the new way to remain a child and stay at home. Those who don't remain dependent by abusing hard drugs find a more acceptable method in being addicted to food as their drug of choice. It is a way to avoid growing up. The hardest relationship to renegotiate will be that between mother and daughter.

"A SON IS A SON 'TILL HE TAKES HIM A WIFE, A DAUGHTER'S A DAUGHTER ALL OF HER LIFE"

From Nancy Friday's *My Mother, Myself* to Collette Dowling's *The Cinderella Complex* and Susie Orbach's *Fat is a Feminist Issue, I and II,* the past decade has produced a plethora of books outlining the struggle between mothers and daughters to separate and develop equality. Many E-D daughters are living out a struggle their parents have not negotiated well. Urged on by Dad to succeed and make him proud, they get the message from Mom that if they don't pursue home and hearth, they are choosing against her and forsaking her values. As a daughter works to gain her mother's approval, Mom only feels defeated and rejected, and thus never approves. It becomes a losing battle.

> *When I began to grow in a different direction, when I left her house, became independent, then conceding my love and admiration of her would have meant an acceptance of beliefs and attitudes which I consider a threat to my existence. . . . During her life I fought her influence, and she fought in me the kind of women who had displaced her.*
>
> Anais Nin, *The Diary of Anais Nin*

When a daughter grows up feeling good about herself, she will probably attract her own mate, marry, and make her own home away from her mother. The current generation of maturing young women are experiencing conflict in this area. By staying fat, women keep mates at bay and don't compete. Adolescent eating disorders signal the woman's inability to leave home. She becomes unable to detach from the nurturance-independence struggle, and thus continues to cling emotionally to Mom, refusing to move out psychologically. This "living at home" exists even if the two reside 3,000 miles apart. As long as the daughter is living more of her life for Mom rather than herself, she is still at home.

Mandy once told me, "I'm not going to O.A.; I hear those people talk and I can tell they want to break up my marriage." Her marriage survived as long as she kept her 350 pounds. This was her second marriage. Her first husband was arrested for drunk driving three times, refused alcoholism treatment and also refused to work. Mandy's mother, Colette, paid off their debts, financed a divorce, and also contributed $3,000 for the intestinal bypass operation which was to save Mandy's life and give her a new start.

Down to 150 pounds, she remarried. Mandy and her mother spent most of every day together while her new husband, Ned, was consumed in his work and getting ahead. As he worked, Mandy and her mother shopped. They also plotted to have a baby. Ned didn't want any more kids; he was supporting two from a previous marriage. Mandy and Colette wanted a child to play with. They also felt it would bring Ned home more and Mandy knew the pregnancy could explain her recently encroaching weight gain. Despite

Ned's protestations, she secretly removed her IUD and a year later gave birth to Jeffrey. She also strayed back up to 350 pounds. Mandy and her mom became engrossed in caring for Jeffrey and talking about dieting. Jeffrey seemed to know his daddy didn't want him, and grew into a hyperactive, raging little boy. Mandy kept eating. She and her mom remained very close. At this juncture I suggested O.A., but she adamantly refused, "for the marriage."

In reality, this marriage was merely a symbol. Mandy was living out a scenario she and Mom had written, and it had nothing to do with Ned. Any guy could have filled the role. Ned knew this and so did little Jeffrey. The significant relationship in this household was between Mandy and her mother. They saw each other daily and shared all their intimacies. Both knew every piece of silverware in the other's drawers as well as every maneuver their partners played in bed. The guys were pawns in the women's game plan. Never could this mother-daughter team say this out loud; they talked instead of male domination and female victimization in the home. Believing they were victims kept them close. Actually, the men had moved out emotionally long ago. One winter Colette went on a cruise, leaving Mandy at home with her husband and son. Within a week, Mandy called me sobbing and immediately attended an O.A. meeting. She said she wanted out of her fat. Two weeks later, they went for family therapy as Jeffrey's acting out became more pronounced. With Mandy's mom out of town, clearly Mandy and Ned faced each other. Little Jeffrey escalated his problem behavior to provide a diversion.

When the cruise ship docked and they drove her mother back home, Mandy stopped going to O.A. and cancelled the next therapy appointment. She feared, "They want to break up my marriage." Actually, there was little in the marriage to break up. Ned worked and complained, Mandy ate and complained, Jeffrey kicked walls and complained. The relationship that had to break up was between mother and daughter. That excessive closeness was defeating the marriage and taking Mandy's life. Instead of negotiating this separation, Mandy and Colette worked out another solution. Colette paid for a second surgical procedure, this time a stomach staple. Mandy's weight is now falling, and Jeffrey is getting worse. We must wait and see what happens when her weight gets down and her spirits pick up. Will she find a way to live her own life, or develop fat or some other problem to keep her close to Mom? Without negotiating the pain of separation, she must continue to suffer to stay close to home.

With support from others in O.A., you will find a way to be close with Mom as well as abstinent. You will learn to risk asking for love instead of settling for food.

Elvira had always had an ideal relationship with her mother, especially after she had her first baby and gained the final 100 of her 360 pounds. She and her mother were never closer than when they shared child rearing stories. Just after the birth, Elvira's younger sister, Natalie, quit smoking. Natalie had always been the "acting out" kid, in contrast to Elvira's "good girl" image. When Natalie quit smoking, excess rage welled to the surface and she began yelling and screaming at her mother every day. To soothe that painful situation, Elvira moved herself right in to be an even better "good girl" so Mommy wouldn't hurt. She and her new infant visited every day. She would stop at the store to prepare for the visit. She appeared each morning with bags full of ice cream, pistachio nuts, popcorn, bagels, noodles, and of course, cottage cheese. With these creations, Elvira set out to be the family mediator. Keeping Mom active in the kitchen kept her out of raging Natalie's path. Mom cooked, Elvira ate. As mediator, she knew just how to tell a joke and turn a phrase to keep her mother and sister from picking at each other. Whenever she got tired or couldn't think of anything to say, she ate. The system worked well until Elvira cut out the excess food. With a committed food plan, the daily visits became more difficult. Elvira didn't know how to listen to the complaints from Mom and younger sister. She also couldn't joke while others were angry. Abstinent, she got more quiet. One day she had to ask her mom for something new.

Mom: So what's wrong with you? You sit around so quietly all the time.

Elvira: I'm just feeling sort of raw since I'm not eating like I used to.

Mom: (She is really missing the good times she used to have when her daughter ate. She feels helpless to make her feel better. She decides to use the family's favorite, time-honored remedy.) Well, I think you're really trying to do too much too fast. Why don't you eat just a little here and there and you'll feel better. I read an article that said it's better to eat many small meals a day instead of waiting for three big meals. Here, have a taste of this pot roast I made and you'll eat less at dinner time.

Elvira: I really want to stick to the food plan I committed to, and I don't want to snack.

Mom: Don't you understand what I'm saying? It's not a snack. You have to get into new ways of thinking with many small meals! You shouldn't have to suffer so much. This O.A. is really making you bitchy!

Elvira: I'm sorry if I'm bitchy, and I can see you really want to help, but I want to follow the direction I'm getting from my sponsor in O.A.

Mom: (Feeling left out and threatened) So who is this sponsor and what does she know? Is she a doctor?

Elvira: No, Ma, it's another person who has been through this and she is instructing me in what she did to lose over 200 pounds.

Mom: Well, everyone is different and I don't think you should be listening to any old nobody in O.A. Why don't you read the article I mentioned and eat like *I* told you?

Discussing how Elvira *should* eat is a way to stay focused on food. Previously, mother and daughter shared recipes, cooked together, and ate while they talked. Now there's a void. The void can be filled with discussions of dieting, but Elvira doesn't want to discuss food at all. She really wants to minimize the importance of food in her life. When food is gone, will there be something else with Mom to take its place?

Elvira: Thanks for your concern, but I'm really trying to find *one* plan and stick to it. I know there are millions of good ideas out there, but if I just find one and stick to it, it won't matter what it is. In the meantime, Mom, let's talk about something else. I'm getting so I really like to stay away from food talk as much as I can.

Mom: (Long silence) So, what should we talk about?

Elvira: (Also quiet, she realizes that it had previously been her responsibility to carry the major direction of family discussion.) I really don't know, Ma. Maybe I just have to be quiet for a while. I'll wait and see.

Mom: (Fearful since her other daughter rages at her most of the time.) I sure wish you'd eat something. I know you'd feel better. I want you should feel better.

Elvira: (Sensing her mother's need for reassurance.) Thanks, Mom. I know you love me. I just need to be quiet and without food for now. I think I'll go home a little early today. I do love you and appreciate you. I could take a nice hug instead of the pot roast.

Since Elvira married, her mother rarely ever touched her. Feeling so close to Elvira, she didn't want to smother her. Mom figured that when Elvira left home to get married, that was the signal to "cut the cord." She set out to stop touching. Her head told her it was best, but her arms ached to hold her "little girl." She offered food as a way to get closer. With food, she was even *inside* her daughter's skin! To Mom, if Elvira wouldn't eat, that meant she didn't accept. Instead, Elvira asked for a hug. She asked for warmth instead of a slab of beef. Mom grabbed her and shook as she held her close. With tears of joy streaming down her face, Elvira wouldn't have taken a doughnut if her life depended on it. She was getting all her needs met in her mother's arms. It's hard to cry and chew at the same time. With joyful hugs, who needs food?

MENACING MENTORS

Those women who move out of the home and kitchen often recreate the mother-daughter dependency in the business world. They may seem to reject their mothers. Most are trying hard to separate, but recreate the struggle on the job. The real separation has to come gently. They have to part as loving friends. A profile of a typical binge vomiter would be a woman 25–35 years old, successful, attractive, with a career in a "man's world," who appears totally self-assured and confident, but is carefully not so successful as to pose a threat. A secret life at home with food keeps this stereotypical victim self-loathing enough not to be too threatening or flying too high.

Wanda was a successful lecturer on management strategies for business. Even though her public valued her expertise, she was still 100 pounds overweight. She was respected by others, but she hated herself. Always in the back of her mind was, "If I'm such a good people manager, why can't I cure myself?" She was sure everyone else thought the same thing. She was also certain that she achieved success because she had really fooled everyone. They would soon find out she was a fraud and had nothing to offer. Despite professional accolades, Wanda believed she was worthless. This attitude kept her fat. Fat is a symbol that something is wrong. It is a warning to others, "Lest you think I may have my act together, take heed first of this enormous bulk of a body and you'll see I still suffer." Wanda did not want to let others see what a truly competent professional she was. She didn't want to believe it herself! As long as she stayed fat, she could postpone living up to her fullest potential. After she lost weight, she quipped, "My potential almost killed me."

Since her basic self-concept was one of inadequacy, Wanda spent many years doubting her professional skills. She remained in her own professional therapy long into recovery. She needed constant validation before she could work. Before giving training seminars, she attended those given by others, comparing herself to them. For many years, she maintained a working contact with a former professor, a powerful mentor, who "had all the answers." She depended on him, a forceful personality who expressed his views with assurance. She found it easy to accept his opinions and reject her own if different. She needed constant reassurance to prove that she was O.K. That relationship worked extremely well; Dr. Gordon liked teaching insecure students who were always questioning and seeking his opinion.

The symbiotic relationship worked, and ultimately all benefited. However, Wanda stayed fat. As her weight loss progressed, she began to feel more confidence in herself and respect for her own views; many of which differed from his. She found his easy, confident answers too superficial. She wanted more complex, careful consideration and thought. She found she had differing professional experience. These changes stressed their relationship. When Dr. Gordon advised her on how to perform professionally, she rebelled by calling him bossy and arrogant. He was shocked! He was just continuing to assume responsibility for her as he had done in the past. She used to like it when he told her what to do and how to act. Wanda didn't need that any more. Since her recovery was progressing, she no longer had fat to keep her down. She was willing to risk being fully who she was; standing for her own opinions. She now needed equal colleagues, not a big daddy. Dr. Gordon felt left out and unnecessary, and actually he was. He was no longer needed. He saw Wanda as arrogant and self-centered. Many heated arguments ensued. The insecure student who had once adoringly sought his guidance, was now rebelling and moving out on her own.

Here were two gifted people who worked helping others. They needed their own help in renegotiating a changed relationship. In her O.A. meetings, Wanda practiced finding a way to lovingly assure her professor that she valued him, but had to grow up and leave him. In the O.A. meetings, she was encouraged to handle the situation in such a way that she would feel good about herself when she walked away. She was to strive for a feeling of well-being, assured that she had not hurt herself or anyone else. If she did not negotiate this well, she might return to bingeing or she might have to continue the dishonest game of pretending she felt inadequate and needy. That was no longer true.

Wanda found that as a recovering person she had a responsibility to consider his feelings as well as her own. When she was the "needy child" she didn't owe him anything, just homage. ("There is no such thing as a free lunch.") Now, since she was a more secure, self-confident adult, she had to consider how her behavior would affect him. She had to be aware of her own strengths and, though scared and shaky herself, she had to think about the other guy. Most of all, she waited until she felt truly loving toward him so she could show him appreciation while breaking away. She had learned at her meetings that "love without honesty is sentimentality, but honesty without love is brutality." At all costs, she had to avoid being brutal. If she felt guilty, she'd punish herself later with food. She wrote the following letter.

Dear Dr. Gordon,

How unfortunate it must be that when you have been outstandingly terrific at teaching and training, you eventually work yourself out of a job! I sure have difficulty giving up feeling needy around you. I still value your pearls of wisdom and well-heeled answers for complex problems.

Unfortunately for us, you taught me a great lesson. It has developed me into a valued professional. You taught

This time, welcome your former self into your new life with love and respect. After all, that poor little kid helped you out of a lot of tough scrapes. That is the person whose best efforts walked you right up to the threshold of this new life. It can't be all bad. It, too, deserves the chance to fly.

As you advance in the O.A. program, you will be encouraged to work with newcomers and help them gain serenity. You may in turn become a sponsor and help reparent a newcomer. In essence, this action is a way for you to heal the wounds of your own childhood. Each time you offer understanding and support to the newcomer, it is a chance for you to give to your own "suffering kid" the things that were missed. In that way, you keep reparenting yourself and welcoming your former self into your new life. That suffering kid has to be laid to rest gently, and with love, so it won't rise up and rebel in fear of flying.

With a gentle, nudging welcome, your sick suffering self won't devour you in recovery. Instead, you will have joined *all* your forces and let the kid come along for the ride. You don't want to throw away the baby with the bath water. Instead, you will bring along the strength that helped you survive the past as well as the super strength you get at O.A. What an unbeatable combination! Good luck, and God bless. . . .